W9-AYN-456

Workbook to Accompany

Cardiopulmonary Anatomy and Physiology

Essentials for Respiratory Care

Fifth Edition

Workbook to Accompany

Cardiopulmonary Anatomy and Physiology

Essentials for Respiratory Care

Fifth Edition

Terry Des Jardins, M.Ed., R.R.T.

Professor Emeritus
Director
Department of Respiratory Care
Parkland College
Champaign, Illinois

THOMSON

DELMAR LEARNING

Australia Brazil Canada Mexico Singapore Spain United Kingdom United States

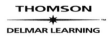

THOMSON

DELMAR LEARNING

Workbook to Accompany Cardiopulmonary Anatomy and Physiology, Essentials for Respiratory Care, 5/e
by Terry Des Jardins

Vice President, Health Care Business Unit:
William Brottmiller

Director of Learning Solutions:
Matthew Kane

Senior Acquisitions Editor:
Rhonda Dearborn

Product Manager:
Sarah Prime

Marketing Director:
Jennifer McAvey

Marketing Coordinator:
Andrea Eobstel

Production Director:
Carolyn Miller

Senior Art Director:
Jack Pendleton

Senior Content Project Manager:
James Zayicek

Technology Product Manager:
Mary Colleen Liburdi

Technology Project Manager:
Carolyn Fox

Library of Congress Card Catalog Number: 2007017383

ISBN 10: 1-4180-4282-X
ISBN 13: 978-1-4180-4282-0

NOTICE TO THE READER

Publisher does not warrant or guarantee any of the products described herein or perform any independent analysis in connection with any of the product information contained herein. Publisher does not assume, and expressly disclaims, any obligation to obtain and include information other than that provided to it by the manufacturer.

The reader is expressly warned to consider and adopt all safety precautions that might be indicated by the activities described herein and to avoid all potential hazards. By following the instructions contained herein, the reader willingly assumes all risks in connection with such instructions.

The publisher makes no representations or warranties of any kind, including but not limited to, the warranties of fitness for particular purpose or merchantability, nor are any such representations implied with respect to the material set forth herein, and the publisher takes no responsibility with respect to such material. The publisher shall not be liable for any special, consequential, or exemplary damages resulting, in whole or part, from the reader's use of, or reliance upon, this material.

CONTENTS

Introduction   vii

Section I / The Cardiopulmonary System—The Essentials   1

Chapter One / The Anatomy and Physiology of the Respiratory System   1

Chapter Two / Ventilation   25

Chapter Three / The Diffusion of Pulmonary Gases   41

Chapter Four / Pulmonary Function Measurements   49

Chapter Five / The Anatomy and Physiology of the Circulatory System   57

Chapter Six / Oxygen Transport   77

Chapter Seven / Carbon Dioxide Transport and Acid-Base Balance   99

Chapter Eight / Ventilation-Perfusion Relationships   129

Chapter Nine / Control of Ventilation   133

Chapter Ten / Fetal Development and the Cardiopulmonary System   139

Chapter Eleven / Aging and the Cardiopulmonary System   149

Section II / Advanced Cardiopulmonary Concepts and Related Areas—The Essentials   153

Chapter Twelve / Electrophysiology of the Heart   153

Chapter Thirteen / The Standard 12-ECG System   157

Chapter Fourteen / ECG Interpretation   163

Chapter Fifteen / Hemodynamic Measurements   183

Chapter Sixteen / Renal Failure and Its Effects
  on the Cardiopulmonary System   191

Chapter Seventeen / Sleep Physiology and Its Relationship   201
  to the Cardiopulmonary System

**Section III / The Cardiopulmonary System During Unusual   211
  Environmental Conditions**

Chapter Eighteen / Exercise and Its Effects on the Cardiopulmonary System   211

Chapter Nineteen / High Altitude and Its Effects on the Cardiopulmonary System   219

Chapter Twenty / High-Pressure Environments and Their Effects   223
  on the Cardiopulmonary System

Answers to Chapter Exercises   227

  Chapter One   228

  Chapter Two   232

  Chapter Three   236

  Chapter Four   238

  Chapter Five   240

  Chapter Six   246

  Chapter Seven   251

  Chapter Eight   257

  Chapter Nine   259

  Chapter Ten   261

  Chapter Eleven   264

  Chapter Twelve   266

  Chapter Thirteen   268

  Chapter Fourteen   271

  Chapter Fifteen   279

  Chapter Sixteen   281

  Chapter Seventeen   284

  Chapter Eighteen   288

  Chapter Nineteen   291

  Chapter Twenty   292

INTRODUCTION

This workbook is designed to enhance the learner's understanding, retention, and clinical application of the material presented in the textbook. The questions in the workbook parallel (in a step-by-step fashion) the information presented in the textbook. The student is asked to do such things as label and color illustrations, fill in the blanks, define terms, match answers, calculate equations, and write short answers.

The completed study questions serve as an excellent study tool to help the student review and prepare for chapter quizzes and exams. This workbook also gives the reader an opportunity to evaluate the degree of mastery of the material presented in the text. Although answering 75 percent of the questions correctly is considered an acceptable mastery level, study and review should continue until greater than 90 percent accuracy has been achieved. The student may wish to copy and maintain unanswered questions of various sections of the workbook for reuse and periodic self-assessment.

Terry Des Jardins

Section I
THE CARDIOPULMONARY SYSTEM— THE ESSENTIALS

CHAPTER ONE

THE ANATOMY AND PHYSIOLOGY OF THE RESPIRATORY SYSTEM

THE UPPER AIRWAY

1. Label and color the following structures of the **upper airway**:

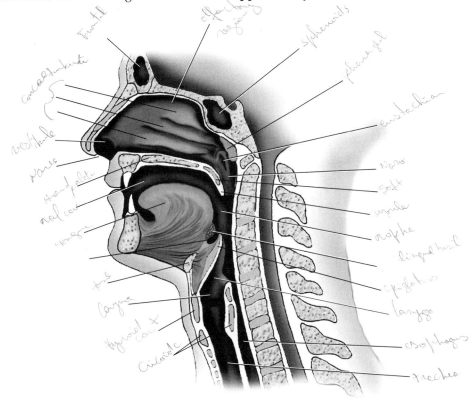

Figure 1-1 *Sagittal section of human head, showing the upper airway.*

2. The primary function(s) of the upper airway are:

   a. ___Conduct gas_____

   _____

   b. ___Prevent aspiration_____

   _____

   c. ___Speech, phonation_____

   _____

   d. ___Olfact smell_____

   _____Humidify, warmth filter gross_____

3. The primary functions of the **nose** are to do the following to inspired air:

   a. ___humidified_____

   b. ___filter_____

   c. ___Smell_____

4. Label and color the following structures that form the outer portion of the nose:

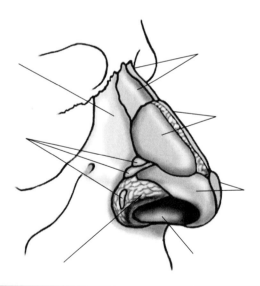

Figure 1–2   *Structure of the nose.*

5. Label and color the following structures of the internal portion of the nose:

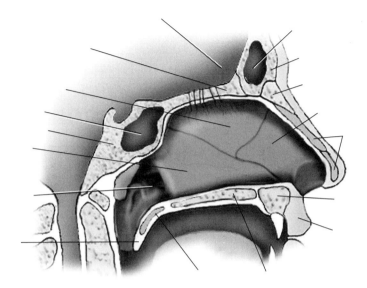

Figure 1–3 *Sagittal section through the nose, showing the parts of the nasal septum.*

6. _____ epithelium lines the posterior two-thirds of the nasal cavity.

7. List the three bony protrusions in the nasal cavity that increase the contact time between the inspired air and the warm, moist surface of the nasal cavity:

a. _____

b. _____

c. _____

8. Label and color the following **sinuses** of the skull:

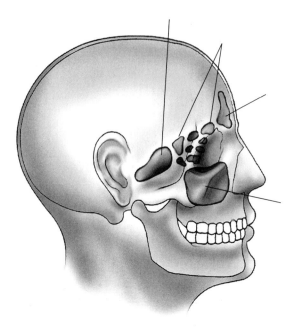

Figure 1–4   *Lateral view of head, showing sinuses.*

9. The _____ muscle elevates the **soft palate**.

10. The **oral cavity** is lined with _____ epithelium.

11. The **palatine arches** are composed of the _____ arch

    and the _____ arch.

12. The **nasopharynx** is lined with ___*Cilied pseudos*_____
epithelium.

13. The ___*estachian tube*_____ serves to equalize the pressure between
the nasopharynx and the middle ear.

14. The **oropharynx** is lined with _____*non ciliated*_____ epithelium.

15. The **laryngopharynx** is lined with _____ epithelium.

16. Label and color the following structures of the oral cavity:

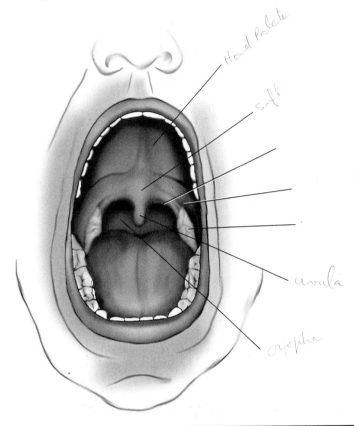

Hard Palate

Soft

uvula

oropha

Figure 1–5 *Oral cavity.*

17. Functionally, the **larynx**:

a. _____

_____

b. _____

_____

c. _____

_____

18. Label and color the structures observed in the superior view of the **vocal folds**:

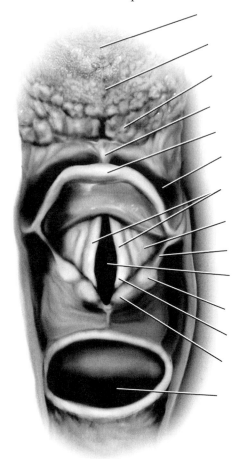

Figure 1–6 *View of the base of the tongue, vallecula epiglottica, epiglottis, and vocal cords.*

19. Label and color the following cartilages of the larynx:

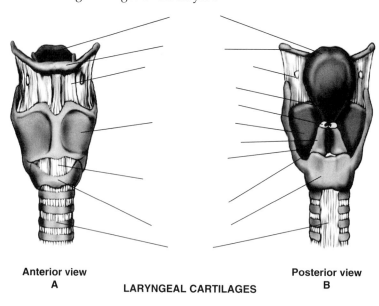

Anterior view
A

LARYNGEAL CARTILAGES

Posterior view
B

Figure 1–7 *Cartilages of the larynx.*

20. The elastic tissue that forms the medial border of each vocal fold is called the _____

    _____ .

21. Anteriorly, the vocal cords attach to the posterior surface of the _____

    _____ .

22. The space between the vocal cords is called the _____ glottis _____

    or the _____ valiala _____ .

23. Above the vocal cords, the laryngeal mucosa is composed of _____

    _____ epithelium.

24. Below the vocal cords, the laryngeal mucosa is lined with _____

    _____ epithelium.

25. An expiratory effort against a closed glottis (e.g., during physical work such as lifting or pushing)

    is known as _____ .

26. Label and color the following **extrinsic laryngeal** muscles:

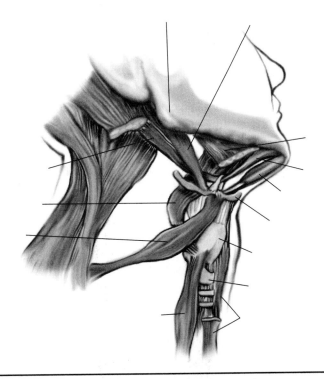

Figure 1–8 *Extrinsic laryngeal muscles.*

27. Label and color the following **intrinsic muscles** of the larynx:

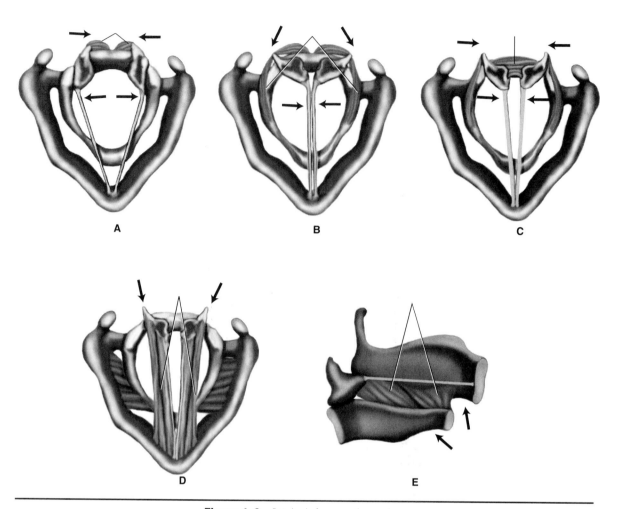

A

B

C

D

E

Figure 1–9   *Intrinsic laryngeal muscles.*

THE LOWER AIRWAYS

1. Label and color the following structures of the tracheobronchial tree:

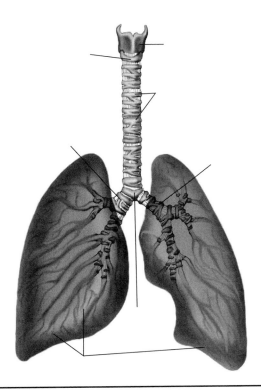

Figure 1–10   *Tracheobronchial tree.*

2. The tracheobronchial tree is composed of the following three layers:

   a. _____

   b. _____

   c. _____

3. The **epithelial lining** of the tracheobronchial tree is mainly composed of _____

   _____ epithelium.

4. Most of the mucous that lines the lumen of the tracheobronchial tree is produced by the

   _____ .

5. The two distinct layers of the mucous blanket are the _____

   and the _____ .

6. Label and color the following section of epithelial lining of the tracheobronchial tree:

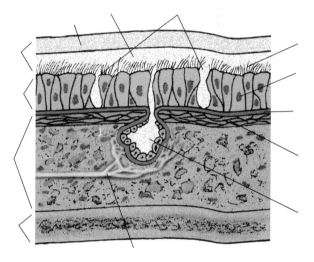

Figure 1–11   *Epithelial lining of the tracheobronchial tree.*

7. List factors that are known to slow the rate of the **mucociliary transport mechanism**:

   a. _____

   b. _____

   c. _____

   d. _____

   e. _____

   f. _____

   g. _____

   h. _____

   i. _____

8. List five chemical mediators of inflammation secreted by the **mast cell**:

a. _____

b. _____

c. _____

d. _____

e. _____

f. _____

9. The adult **trachea** is about _____ to _____ cm long and _____ to _____ cm in diameter.

10. The bifurcation of the trachea is known as the _____.

11. In the adult, the right **main stem bronchus** branches off the vertical trachea at about a _____ -degree angle; the left main stem bronchus forms a _____ to _____ -degree angle with the vertical trachea.

12. **Canals of Lambert** are found in the _____ of the tracheobronchial tree.

13. From the trachea to the **terminal bronchioles**, the total cross-sectional area of the tracheobronchial tree progressively _____ .

14. The **bronchial arteries** nourish the tracheobronchial tree down to, and including, the _____ _____ .

15. In addition to the tracheobronchial tree, the bronchial arteries nourish the

_____

_____

_____

_____

16. Approximately one-third of the bronchial venous blood returns to the right atrium by way of the

_____

_____

17. About two-thirds of the bronchial venous blood empties into the pulmonary circulation by means

    of _____

    _____

THE SITES OF GAS EXCHANGE

1. The anatomic structures distal to the terminal bronchioles consist of the

   a. _____ bronchioles

   b. _____ ducts

   c. _____ sacs

2. Using the following schematic drawing, label the following anatomic structures distal to the terminal bronchiole:

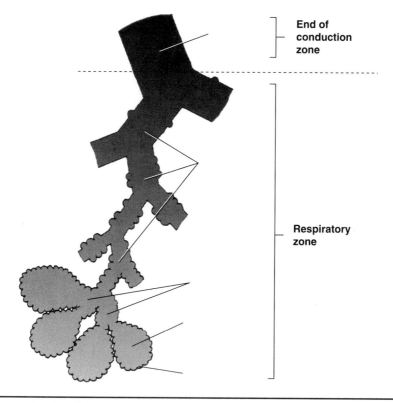

Figure 1–12 *Schematic drawing of the anatomic structures distal to the terminal bronchioles; collectively, these are referred to as the primary lobule.*

3. Label and color the following components of the alveolar-capillary network:

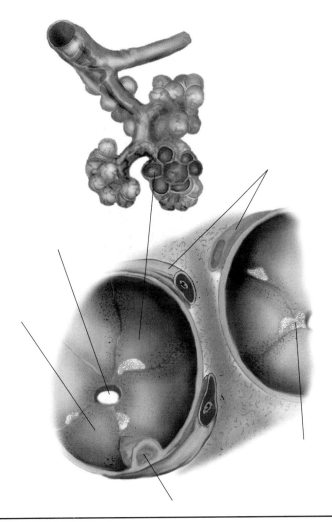

Figure 1–13 *Alveolar-capillary network.*

4. In the adult lung, there are approximately _____ million alveoli.

5. The average surface area of the adult lung is _____ square meters.

6. A **primary lobule** consists of which structures distal to a single terminal bronchiole?

_____

_____

7. There are approximately _____ primary lobules in the lung.

8. Synonyms of a primary lobule are

   a. _____

   b. _____

   c. _____

   d. _____

9. The **type I cell** found in the alveolar epithelium is also called a _____

  _____ .

10. The **type II cell** found in the alveolar epithelium is also called a _____

  _____ .

11. The type I cells form about _____ percent of the alveolar substance.

12. The _____ cells are believed to be the primary source of **pulmonary surfactant**.

13. Small holes in the walls of the interalveolar septa are called _____

  _____ .

14. The _____ play a major role in removing foreign
particles that are deposited within the **acini**.

15. The two major compartments of the **interstitium** are the _____

  and the _____ .

PULMONARY VASCULAR SYSTEM AND LYMPHATIC SYSTEM

1. Using the following schematic drawing, label and color the components of the major blood vessels:

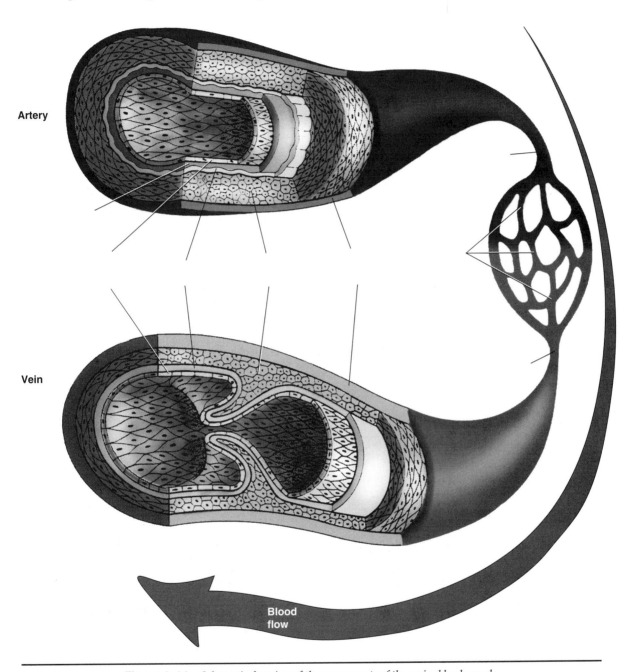

Figure 1–14   *Schematic drawing of the components of the major blood vessels.*

2. The **arterioles** play an important role in the distribution and regulation of blood and are called

   the _____ vessels.

3. The walls of the pulmonary **capillaries** are less than _____ thick and the external

   diameter is about _____ .

4. Because the **veins** are capable of collecting a large amount of blood with very little pressure change,

   the veins are called _____ vessels.

5. Superficially, **lymphatic vessels** are found around the lung just beneath the _____

   _____ .

6. Within the lungs, the lymphatic vessels arise from the _____

   _____ .

7. Label the following **lymph nodes** associated with the trachea and the right and left main stem bronchi:

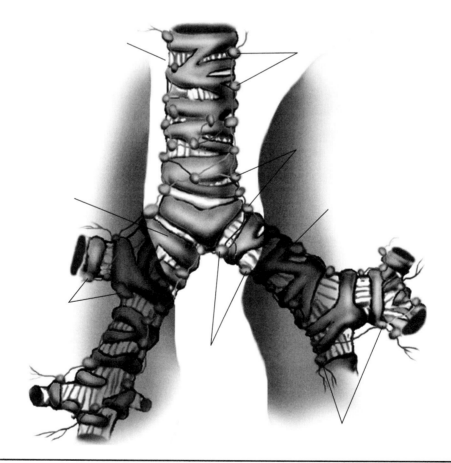

Figure 1–15 *Lymph nodes associated with the trachea and the right and left main stem bronchi.*

NEURAL CONTROL OF THE LUNGS

1. The smooth muscle that surrounds the bronchi and arterioles is controlled by the _____

   _____ .

2. Compare the effects of the **sympathetic** and **parasympathetic nervous system** on the following effector sites:

TABLE 1–1   **Some Effects of Autonomic Nervous System Activity**

EFFECTOR SITE	SYMPATHETIC NERVOUS SYSTEM	PARASYMPATHETIC NERVOUS SYSTEM
Heart		
Bronchial smooth muscle		
Bronchial glands		
Salivary glands		
Stomach		
Intestines		
Eye		

3. When the sympathetic nervous system is activated, _____

   or _____ neural transmitters are released.

4. When the **beta$_2$ receptors** are stimulated, the bronchial smooth muscles _____

   _____ .

5. When the **alpha receptors** are stimulated, the smooth muscles of the arterioles _____

   _____ .

6. When the parasympathetic nervous system is activated, the neural transmitter _____

   _____ is released.

THE LUNGS

1. The apices of the lungs rise to about the level of the _____ rib.

2. Anteriorly, the base of the lungs extends to about the level of the _____ rib, and posteriorly to about the level of the _____ rib.

3. At the center of the **mediastinal border**, the right and left main stem bronchi, blood vessels, lymph vessels, and various nerves enter and exit the lungs through the _____ .

4. In the **right lung**, the **oblique fissure** extends from the _____ to the _____ borders.

5. In the right lung, the **horizontal fissure** extends horizontally from the _____ to about the level of the _____ costal cartilage.

6. In the **left lung**, the oblique fissure extends from the _____ to the _____ borders of the lung.

7. Label the following structures of the anterior portion of the lungs:

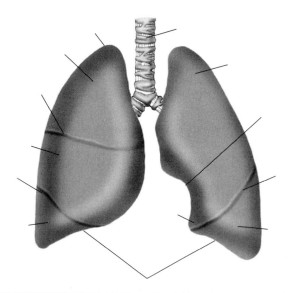

Figure 1–16 *Anterior view of the lungs.*

8. Label the following structures of the medial portion of the lungs:

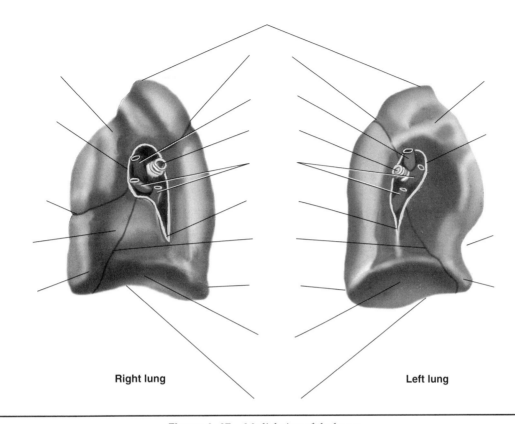

Right lung　　　　　　　　　　　　　　**Left lung**

Figure 1–17 *Medial view of the lungs.*

9. Match the number of the lung segments shown in the box to the different views of the lung. Content retention is also enhanced when the lung segments are colored.

	Right lung			Left lung	
Upper lobe			Upper lobe		
Apical	1		Upper division		
Posterior	2		Apical/Posterior		1 & 2
Anterior	3		Anterior		3
Middle lobe			Lower division (lingular)		
Lateral	4		Superior lingula		4
Medial	5		Inferior lingula		5
Lower lobe			Lower lobe		
Superior	6		Superior		6
Medial basal	7		Anterior medial basal		7 & 8
Anterior basal	8		Lateral basal		9
Lateral basal	9		Posterior basal		10
Posterior basal	10				

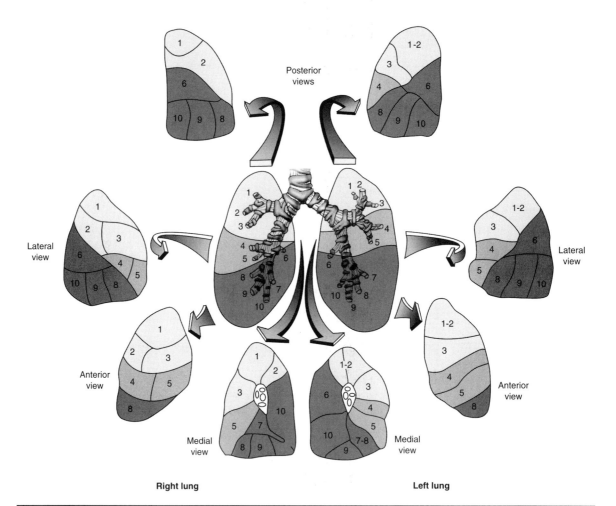

Figure 1–18 *Lung segments. Although the segment subdivisions of the right and left lungs are similar, there are some slight anatomic differences, which are noted by combined names and numbers. Because of these slight variations, some researchers consider that, technically, there are only eight segments in the left lung and that the apical-posterior segment is number 1 and the anteromedial is number 6.*

10. Label the following major structures around the lungs:

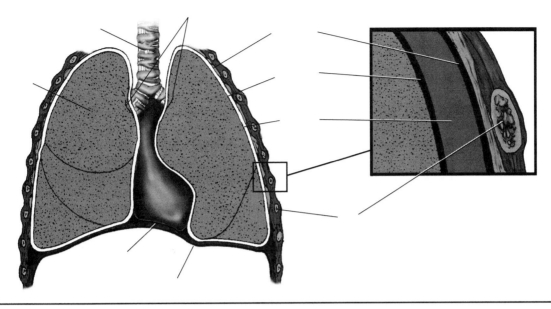

Figure 1–19   *Major structures around the lungs.*

THE MEDIASTINUM, PLEURAL MEMBRANES, AND THORAX

1. List the anatomic structures that are contained in, or pass through, the **mediastinum**:

   _____

   _____

   _____

2. The _____ pleura is firmly attached to the outer surface of each lung.

3. The _____ pleura lines the inside of the thoracic walls.

4. The potential space between the pleural membranes is called the _____

   _____ .

5. List the three major structures that compose the **sternum**:

    a. _____

    b. _____

    c. _____

6. The first seven ribs are called the _____.

7. Ribs eight, nine and ten are referred to as the _____ ribs.

8. Ribs eleven and twelve are called the _____ ribs.

9. Label the following components of the **thorax**:

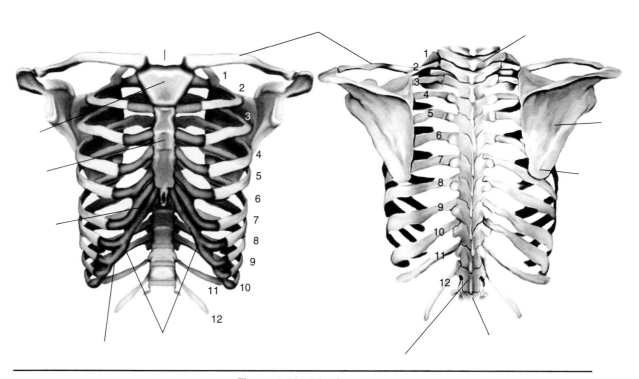

Figure 1–20   *The thorax.*

10. Label the following components of the intercostal space:

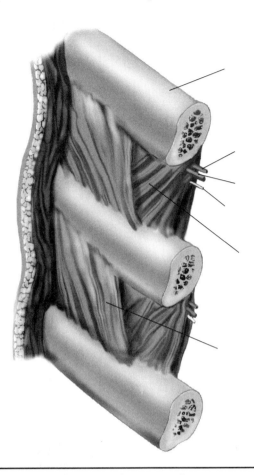

Figure 1–21 *The intercostal space.*

THE DIAPHRAGM

1. Each **hemidiaphragm** merges together at the midline into a broad connective sheet called the

   _____ .

2. List the structures that pierce the **diaphragm**:

   _____

   _____

3. The _____ nerves supply the primary motor innervation to each hemidiaphragm.

4. When used as accessory muscles for inspiration, the **scalenus muscles** elevate the

_____ and _____ ribs.

5. When used as accessory muscles of inspiration, the **sternocleidomastoid muscles** elevate the

_____ .

6. When used as accessory muscles of inspiration, the **pectoralis major muscles** elevate the

_____ , causing an increased _____

diameter.

7. Normally, the **trapezius muscles** rotate the _____ , raise the _____ ,

and abduct and flex the _____ .

8. During inspiration, the **external intercostal muscles** pull the ribs _____ and

_____ .

9. Label and color the following accessory muscles of expiration:

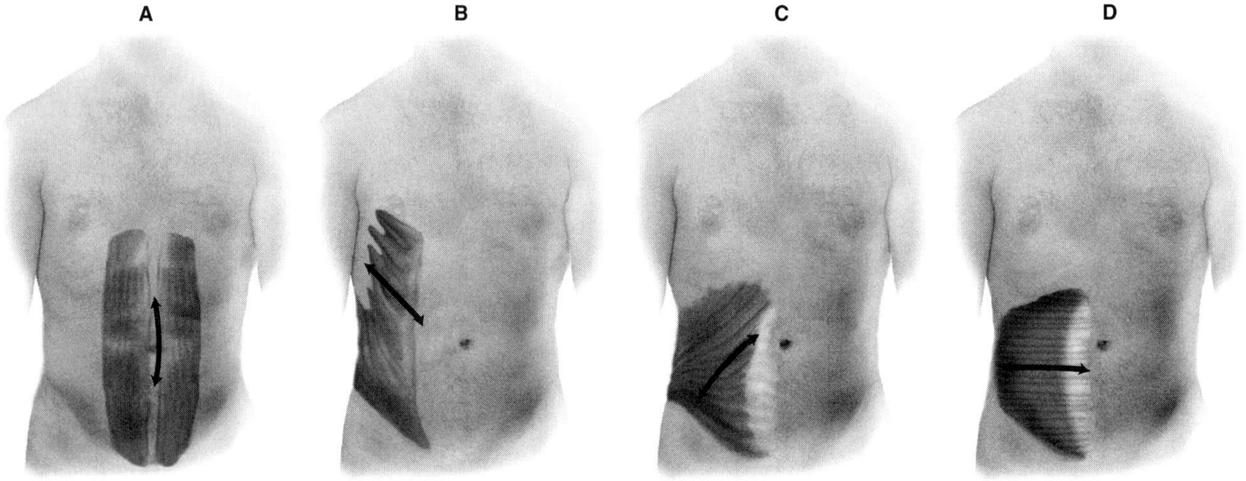

Figure 1–22 *Accessory muscles of expiration.*

10. During exhalation, the **internal intercostal muscles** pull the ribs _____ and

_____ .

CHAPTER TWO

VENTILATION

PRESSURE DIFFERENCES ACROSS THE LUNGS

1. The pressure difference between two points in a tube or vessel is called the _____ _____ .

2. The barometric pressure difference between the mouth pressure and alveolar pressure is called the _____ .

3. When the pressure is greater within the airway, the pressure is called _____ _____ .

4. When the pressure is greater outside the airway, the pressure is called _____ _____ .

5. The difference between the alveolar pressure and the pleural pressure is called the _____ _____ .

6. The difference between the alveolar pressure and the body surface pressure is called the _____ .

7. If the gas pressure at the beginning of a vessel is 12 mm Hg and the pressure at the other end of the same vessel is 7 mm Hg, what is the driving pressure?

Answer: _____

8. If the P_{alv} is 751 mm Hg and the P_m is 758 mm Hg, what is the P_{ta}?

Answer: _____

9. If the P_{pl} is 752 mm Hg and the P_{alv} is 748 mm Hg, what is the P_{tp}?

Answer: _____

10. If the P_{alv} is 751 mm Hg and the P_{bs} is 757 mm Hg, what is the P_{tt}?

Answer: _____

11. During inspiration, the thoracic volume increases and the intrapleural and intra-alveolar pressures

_____ .

12. During expiration, the intra-alveolar pressure is (_____ greater; _____ lower) than the barometric pressure.

13. During a normal expiration, the intrapleural pressure is always (_____ above; _____ below) the barometric pressure.

14. The normal intrapleural pressure change is about _____ to _____ cm H_2O pressure, or _____

to _____ mm Hg.

ELASTIC PROPERTIES OF THE LUNG AND CHEST WALL

1. **Lung compliance** is defined as the change in lung _____ per change in _____

   _____ .

2. **Case A**

   a. If an individual generates an intrapleural pressure of -7 cm H_2O during inspiration, and the lungs accept a new volume of 385 ml of air, what is the compliance of the lungs?

   Answer: _____

   b. If the same patient, four hours later, generates an intrapleural pressure of -5 cm H_2O during inspiration, and the lungs accept a new volume of 350 ml of air, what is the compliance of the lungs?

   Answer: _____

   c. The lung compliance of the above patient is (increasing _____ ; decreasing _____).

3. **Case B**

   a. If a mechanical ventilator generates a $+9$ cm H_2O pressure during inspiration and the lungs accept a new volume of 450 ml of gas, what is the compliance of the lungs?

   Answer: _____

b. If, on the same patient six hours later, the mechanical ventilator generates a +15 cm H_2O pressure and the lungs accept a new volume of 675 ml of gas, what is the compliance of the lungs?

Answer: _____

c. Compare the answers to the first two questions (a & b). The patient's lung compliance is (increasing _____ ; decreasing _____).

4. Under normal resting conditions, the average lung compliance during each breath is approximately

_____ .

5. According to the volume-pressure curve (Figure 2-1), if an individual has a resting lung volume of 1500 ml, and generates a negative 25 cm H_2O pressure (in addition to the negative pressure required to maintain the resting lung volume), how many ml of gas will the lungs accommodate (in addition to the resting lung volume)?

Answer: _____

6. When lung compliance decreases, the volume-pressure curve moves to the _____ .

7. When the volume-pressure curve moves to the left, lung compliance is (circle one):
   a. increased
   b. decreased
   c. unchanged

8. As the alveoli approach their total filling capacity, lung compliance:
   a. increases
   b. decreases
   c. remains the same

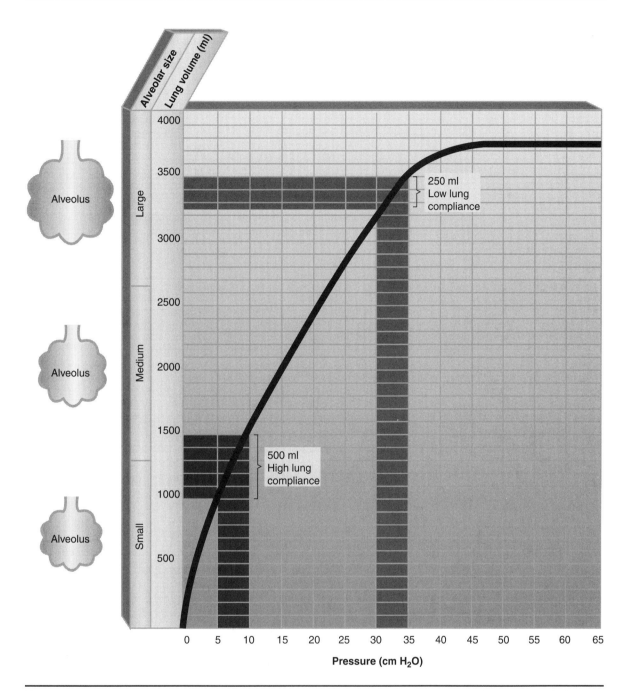

Figure 2–1   *Normal volume-pressure curve. The curve shows that lung compliance progressively decreases as the lungs expand in response to more volume. For example, note the greater volume change between 5 and 10 cm H_2O (small/medium alveoli) than between 30 and 35 cm H_2O (large alveoli).*

9. **Elastance** is defined as _____

_____

_____

_____

_____

_____

10. In pulmonary physiology, elastance is defined as _____ and is expressed as:

Elastance =

11. Lungs with high compliance have _____ elastance, and lungs with low compliance

have _____ elastance.

12. **Hooke's law** states that _____

_____

_____

_____

_____

_____ .

13. When Hooke's law is applied to the elastic properties of the lungs, _____ is

substituted for *length* and _____ is substituted for *force*.

14. The molecular, cohesive force at the liquid–gas interface is called _____ .

15. The liquid film that lines the interior surface of the alveoli has the potential to exert a force of

_____ .

16. When Laplace's law is applied to a sphere with one liquid–gas interface, the equation is written as follows:

P =

17. The mathematical arrangement of Laplace's law shows that the distending pressure of a liquid bubble is

    a. _____

    _____

    and

    b. _____

    _____ .

18. According to Laplace's law, as the surface tension of a liquid bubble increases, the distending pressure required to hold the bubble open _____ ; and as the radius of the bubble increases, the distending pressure _____ .

19. When two different-sized bubbles with the same surface tension are in direct communication the
    a. larger bubble will empty into the smaller bubble
    b. smaller bubble will empty into the larger bubble
    c. distending pressures in the two bubbles are equal; thus there is no gas flow between the two bubbles.

20. During the formation of a new bubble, the principles of Laplace's law do not come into effect until the distending pressure of the liquid sphere goes beyond the _____ .

21. As a liquid bubble increases in size, the surface tension
    a. increases
    b. decreases
    c. remains the same

22. **Pulmonary surfactant** is produced by the _____ .

23. The surfactant molecule has both a hydrophobic end, which means it is _____ , and a hydrophilic end, which means it is _____ .

24. In the healthy lung, when the alveolus decreases in size, the amount of surfactant to alveolar surface area _____ . This action causes the alveolar surface tension to _____

    _____ .

25. It is estimated that the surface tension of the average alveolus varies from _____ in the small alveolus to about _____ in the fully distended alveolus.

26. List some general causes of surfactant deficiency:

    a. _____

    b. _____

    c. _____

    d. _____

    e. _____

27. In the healthy lung, both the elastic force and the surface tension force are (_____ low; _____ high) in the small alveolus.

DYNAMIC CHARACTERISTICS OF THE LUNGS

1. The term **dynamic** is defined as the _____

   _____

2. In the lungs, dynamic refers to _____

   _____

3. When Poiseuille's law is arranged for flow $\dot{V}$, it is written as follows:

   $\dot{V} =$

4. According to Poiseuille's law, and assuming all other variables remain the same,

   a. as the pressure increases, flow (_____ increases; _____ decreases)

   b. as the length of a tube decreases, flow (_____ increases; _____ decreases)

   c. as the radius of a tube increases, flow (_____ increases; _____ decreases)

   d. as the viscosity decreases, flow (_____ increases; _____ decreases)

5. Using Poiseuille's law equations and assuming all other variables remain the same, answer the following questions:

   a. If the radius of a tube that has gas flowing through it at 32 liters per minute (L/min) is reduced by 50 percent of its original size, what will be the new gas flow through the tube?

      Answer: _____

b. If the radius of a tube that has gas flowing through it at 28 L/min is reduced by 16 percent, what will be the new gas flow through the tube?

Answer: _____

c. If the radius of a tube that has a driving pressure of 16 cm H_2O is reduced by 50 percent of its original size, what will be the new driving pressure required to maintain the same gas flow through the tube?

Answer: _____

d. If the radius of a tube that has a driving pressure of 10 cm H_2O is reduced by 16 percent of its original size, what will be the new driving pressure required to maintain the same gas flow through the tube?

Answer: _____

e. If the radius of a tube that has gas flowing through it at 160 L/min is decreased by 50 percent of its original size, what will be the new gas flow through the tube?

Answer: _____

f. If the radius of a tube that has gas flowing through it at 100 L/min is decreased by 16 percent of its original size, what will be the new gas flow through the tube?

Answer: _____

g. If the radius of a tube that has a driving pressure of 10 cm H_2O is decreased by 50 percent of its original size, what will be the new driving pressure required to maintain the same gas flow through the tube?

Answer: _____

h. If the radius of a tube that has a driving pressure of 5 cm H_2O is decreased by 16 percent of its original size, what will be the new driving pressure required to maintain the same gas flow through the tube?

Answer: _____

6. Write the simple proportionalities of Poiseuille's law for flow ($\dot{V}$) and pressure (P):

$\dot{V} =$

$P =$

AIRWAY RESISTANCE AND DYNAMIC COMPLIANCE

1. Airway resistance (R_{aw}) is defined as the _____

   _____

   _____

2. Write the equation for airway resistance (R_{aw}) and include the units of measurement:

   R_{aw} =

3. If a patient produces a flow rate of 10 liters per second (L/sec) during inspiration by generating a transairway pressure (P_{ta}) of 30 cm H_2O, what is the patient's R_{aw}?

   Answer: _____

4. The normal R_{aw} in the tracheobronchial tree is about _____ to _____ cm H_2O/L/sec.

5. Laminar gas flow refers to _____

   _____

6. Turbulent gas flow refers to _____

   _____

7. Time constant is defined as the _____

   _____

   _____

8. Lung regions that have an increased airway resistance require
   a. less time to inflate
   b. more time to inflate
   c. no change in time to inflate

9. Lung regions that have an increased compliance require
   a. less time to inflate
   b. more time to inflate
   c. no change in time to inflate

10. Which of the following causes lung regions to have a long time constant?
    I. decreased airway resistance
    II. increased lung compliance
    III. increased airway resistance
    IV. decreased lung compliance
       a. I only
       b. III only
       c. II and III only
       d. III and IV only
       e. II, III, and IV only

11. Lung regions that have a decreased airway resistance require
    a. less time to inflate
    b. more time to inflate
    c. no change in time to inflate

12. Lung regions that have a decreased compliance require
    a. less time to inflate
    b. more time to inflate
    c. no change in time to inflate

13. Which of the following causes lung regions to have a short time constant?
    I. increased airway resistance
    II. decreased lung compliance
    III. decreased airway resistance
    IV. increased lung compliance
       a. II only
       b. IV only
       c. III only
       d. I and IV only
       e. II and III only

14. **Dynamic compliance** is defined as the _____

    _____

    _____

    _____

15. In the normal lung, the dynamic compliance is (_____ equal to; _____ greater than; _____ less than) lung compliance at all breathing frequencies.

16. In the partially obstructed airways, the ratio of dynamic compliance to lung compliance (_____ increases; _____ decreases; _____ remains the same) as the breathing frequency increases.

17. Frequency dependent refers to _____

_____

_____

_____

_____

VENTILATORY PATTERNS

1. The ventilatory pattern consists of the following three components:

   a. _____

   b. _____

   c. _____

2. The normal **tidal volume** is about _____ to _____ mL/kg; or _____ to _____ mL/lb.

3. The normal adult ventilatory rate is about _____ breaths per minute.

4. The normal I : E is about _____ : _____.

5. The gas that reaches the alveoli during inspiration is referred to as _____.

6. The gas that does not reach the alveoli during inspiration is referred to as _____

_____.

7. **Anatomic dead space** is defined as _____

_____

_____

_____

8. If a patient weighs 130 pounds, about how many milliliters (mL) of inspired gas during each breath would be anatomic dead space gas?

Answer: _____

9. **Alveolar ventilation** is equal to the _____ minus the _____

multiplied by the _____ .

10. An individual presents with this data:

   - V_T = 575 mL
   - V_D = 185 mL
   - Breaths/minute = 16

What is the alveolar ventilation?

Answer: _____

11. **Alveolar dead space** is defined as _____

_____

_____

12. **Physiologic dead space** is defined as _____

_____

13. In the upright position, the negative intrapleural pressure at the apex of the lung is normally (_____

less; _____ greater) than at the base.

14. In the upright position, the alveoli in the upper lung regions are (_____ smaller; _____ larger;

_____ equal) in size compared to the alveoli in the lower lung regions.

15. In the upright lung, ventilation is much greater in the
    a. upper lung regions
    b. middle lung regions
    c. lower lung regions

16. When lung compliance decreases, the patient's ventilatory rate generally (_____ increases; _____ decreases; _____ remains the same) and the tidal volume (_____ increases; _____ decreases; _____ remains the same).

17. When airway resistance increases, the patient's ventilatory rate generally (_____ increases; _____ decreases; _____ remains the same) and the tidal volume (_____ increases; _____ decreases; _____ remains the same) .

18. In response to a certain respiratory disorder, the patient may adopt a ventilatory pattern based on the expenditure of _____ rather than the efficiency of _____ .

19. **Apnea** is defined as the _____

20. **Eupnea** is defined as _____

21. **Biot's breathing** is defined as _____

22. **Hyperpnea** is defined as _____

23. **Hyperventilation** is defined as _____

_____

_____

_____

24. **Hypoventilation** is defined as _____

_____

_____

_____

25. **Tachypnea** is defined as _____

_____

26. **Cheyne-Stokes breathing** is defined as _____

_____

_____

_____

_____

27. **Kussmaul breathing** is defined as _____

_____

_____

28. **Orthopnea** is defined as _____

_____

_____

_____

29. **Dyspnea** is defined as _____

_____

_____

CHAPTER THREE

THE DIFFUSION
OF PULMONARY GASES

DIFFUSION AND GAS LAWS

1. **Diffusion** is defined as _____

_____

_____

2. Boyle's law states that _____

_____

_____

3. Boyle's law is written as follows:

4. If an airtight container which has a volume of 400 mL and a pressure of 50 cm H_2O has its volume reduced to 300 mL, what will be the new pressure in the container?

Answer: _____

5. If an airtight container which has a volume of 55 mL and a pressure of 75 cm H_2O has its volume increased to 110 mL, what will be the new pressure in the container?

Answer: _____

6. Charles' law states that _____

_____

_____

_____

7. Charles' law is written as follows:

8. If the temperature of gas in an 8-liter balloon is increased from 290 Kelvin to 340 Kelvin, what will be the new volume in the balloon?

Answer: _____

9. If the temperature of an automobile tire which has 4.5 liters of air in it is increased from 32° Celsius to 42° Celsius, what will be the new volume of gas (air) in the tire?

Answer: _____

10. Gay-Lussac's law states that _____

_____

_____

_____

11. Gay-Lussac's law is written as follows:

12. If the temperature of gas in a closed container which has a pressure of 15 cm H_2O is increased from 360 Kelvin to 375 Kelvin, what will be the new pressure in the container?

Answer: _____

13. If the temperature of the gas in a closed container which has a pressure of 46 cm H_2O is decreased from 40° Celsius to 30° Celsius, what will be the new pressure in the container?

Answer: _____

14. Dalton's law states that _____

_____

_____

_____

15. The following gases and their respective pressures are enclosed in a container:

GAS	PARTIAL PRESSURE
Nitrogen	470 mm Hg
Oxygen	130 mm Hg
Carbon Dioxide	50 mm Hg

According to Dalton's law, what is the total pressure in the container?

Answer: _____

THE PARTIAL PRESSURES OF ATMOSPHERIC GASES

1. At sea level, identify the percentage of the atmosphere and the partial pressure of the following gases that compose the barometric pressure:

TABLE 3–1   Gases That Compose the Barometric Pressure

GAS	% OF ATMOSPHERE	PARTIAL PRESSURE (mm Hg)
Nitrogen (N_2)		
Oxygen (O_2)		
Argon (Ar)		
Carbon dioxide (CO_2)		

2. As one ascends a mountain, the barometric pressure (_____ increases; _____ decreases; _____ remains the same) and the percent concentration of oxygen (_____ increases; _____ decreases; _____ remains the same).

3. Compare the partial pressure of gases in the dry air, alveoli, arterial blood, and venous blood:

TABLE 3–2   Partial Pressure (in mm Hg) of Gases in the Air, Alveoli, and Blood

GASES	DRY AIR	ALVEOLAR GAS	ARTERIAL BLOOD	VENOUS BLOOD
P_{O_2}				
P_{CO_2}				
P_{H_2O} (water vapor)				
P_{N_2} (and other gases in minute quantities)				
Total				

4. The reason the partial pressure of oxygen in the atmosphere is so much higher than the partial pressure of oxygen in the alveoli is because

_____

_____

_____

_____

5. At body temperature, the alveolar gas has an absolute humidity of _____ and a water

   vapor pressure (P_{H_2O}) of _____ .

6. If a patient is receiving an FI_{O_2} of 0.70 on a day when the barometric pressure is 748 mm Hg, and if the Pa_{CO_2} is 50 mm Hg, what is the patient's alveolar oxygen tension (PA_{O_2})?

   Answer: _____

THE DIFFUSION OF PULMONARY GASES

1. List the structures of the alveolar-capillary membrane that gas molecules must diffuse through:

   a. _____

   b. _____

   c. _____

   d. _____

   e. _____

   f. _____

   g. _____

   h. _____

   i. _____

2. The thickness of the alveolar-capillary membrane is between _____ and

   _____ .

3. In the healthy resting person, the average $P\bar{v}_{O_2}$ is _____ mm Hg and the average $P\bar{v}_{CO_2}$ is

   _____ mm Hg.

4. Under normal circumstances, when venous blood enters the alveolar-capillary system, there is an

   oxygen pressure gradient of about _____ mm Hg, and a carbon dioxide pressure gradient of

   about _____ mm Hg.

5. The equilibrium of oxygen and carbon dioxide in the alveolar-capillary system is usually accom-

   plished in about _____ second.

6. The total transit time for blood to move through the alveolar-capillary system is about

   _____ second, which is about _____ of the time available.

7. During exercise, the time available for gas diffusion (circle one)

   a. increases
   b. decreases
   c. remains the same

8. Fick's law is written as follows:

   $\dot{V}$ gas $\propto$

9. According to Fick's law, as the
   a. thickness decreases, gas diffusion (circle one)

      a. increases
      b. decreases
      c. remains the same

   b. pressure difference increases, gas diffusion

      a. increases
      b. decreases
      c. remains the same

   c. area decreases, gas diffusion

      a. increases
      b. decreases
      c. remains the same

10. Henry's law states that _____

_____

_____

_____ .

11. The amount of gas that can be dissolved by 1 mL of a given liquid at standard pressure and speci-

fied temperature is known as the _____ .

12. Graham's law states that the rate of diffusion of a gas through a liquid is

a. _____

_____

_____

and

b. _____

_____ .

PERFUSION- AND DIFFUSION-LIMITED GAS FLOW

1. **Perfusion limited** means that _____

_____

_____

_____

2. **Diffusion limited** means that _____

_____

_____

_____

3. Under normal circumstances, the diffusion of oxygen is
    a. perfusion limited
    b. diffusion limited
    c. neither perfusion nor diffusion limited

CHAPTER FOUR

PULMONARY FUNCTION MEASUREMENTS

LUNG VOLUMES AND CAPACITIES

1. **Tidal volume** (V_T) is defined as _____

   _____

   _____

2. **Inspiratory reserve volume** (IRV) is defined as _____

   _____

   _____

3. **Expiratory reserve volume** (ERV) is defined as _____

   _____

   _____

4. **Residual volume** (RV) is defined as _____

   _____

   _____

5. **Vital capacity** (VC) is defined as _____

   _____

   _____

6. **Inspiratory capacity (IC) is defined as** _____

   _____

   _____

7. **Functional residual capacity (FRC) is defined as** _____

   _____

   _____

8. **Total lung capacity (TLC) is defined as** _____

   _____

   _____

9. **Residual volume/total lung capacity ratio (RV/TLC × 100) is defined as** _____

   _____

   _____

10. Compare the approximate lung volumes and capacities in the average normal male and female between 20 and 30 years of age:

TABLE 4–1   **Approximate Lung Volumes and Capacities in Healthy Men and Women 20 to 30 Years of Age**

	MEN		WOMEN	
MEASUREMENT	**mL**	**Approx. % of TLC**	**mL**	**Approx. % of TLC**
Tidal volume (V_T)				
Inspiratory reserve volume (IRV)				
Expiratory reserve volume (ERV)				
Residual volume (RV)				
Vital capacity (VC)				
Inspiratory capacity (IC)				
Functional residual capacity (FRC)				
Total lung capacity (TLC)				
Residual volume/Total lung capacity ratio (RV/TLC × 100)				

11. In an obstructive lung disorder, the _____ , _____ , _____ , and _____ are increased; and the _____ , _____ , _____ , and _____ are decreased.

12. In a restrictive lung disorder, the _____ , _____ , _____ , _____ , _____ , and _____ are all decreased.

13. Because the *residual volume* (RV) cannot be exhaled, the RV, and lung capacities that contain the RV, are measured indirectly by one of the following methods:

    a. _____

    b. _____

    c. _____

PULMONARY MECHANICS

1. **Forced vital capacity** (FVC) is defined as _____

   _____

   _____

   _____

2. **Forced expiratory volume timed** (FEV_T) is defined as _____

   _____

   _____

3. The normal percentage of the total volume exhaled during the following time periods is

   a. $FEV_{0.5}$ _____ percent

   b. $FEV_{1.0}$ _____ percent

   c. $FEV_{2.0}$ _____ percent

   d. $FEV_{3.0}$ _____ percent

4. In obstructive disease, the percentage of FVC that can be forcefully exhaled over a specific period of time (_____ increases; _____ decreases; _____ remains the same).

5. Forced expiratory volume$_{1\,Sec}$/Forced vital capacity ratio (FEV_1/FVC ratio) is the _____

   _____

6. Because the FEV_1/FVC ratio is expressed as a percentage, it is commonly referred to as a _____

   _____

7. Under normal conditions the patient's $FEV_{1\%}$ shoud be _____ or greater.

8. Collectively, the FEV, FEV_1, and the $FEV_{1\%}$ are the most commonly used pulmonary function measurements to

   a. _____

   b. _____

9. In obstructive lung disorders, both the FEV_1 and the $FEV_{1\%}$ are (_____ decreased; _____ increased).

10. In restrictive lung disorders, the FEV_1 is down, but the $FEV_{1\%}$ is _____ .

11. **Forced expiratory flow$_{25\%-75\%}$** ($FEF_{25\%-75\%}$) is defined as _____

    _____

    _____

    _____

12. The $FEF_{25\%-75\%}$ reflects the status of the _____ to _____ -sized airways.

13. **Forced expiratory flow$_{200-1200}$** ($FEF_{200-1200}$) is defined as _____

    _____

    _____

    _____

14. The $FEF_{200-1200}$ is a good index of the (_____ large; _____ small) airway function.

15. **Peak expiratory flow rate** (PEFR) is defined as _____

    _____

    _____

16. **Maximum voluntary ventilation** (MVV) is defined as _____

    _____

    _____

17. Label the following measurements graphically presented in the **flow-volume loop**:

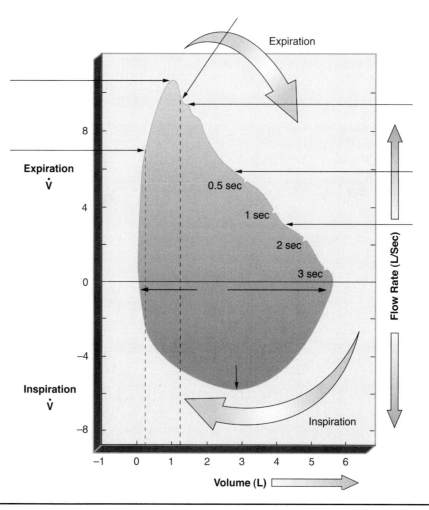

Figure 4–1 *Normal flow-volume loop.*

18. Compare the following average dynamic flow rate measurements of the healthy male and female between 20 and 30 years of age:

TABLE 4–2   **Average Dynamic Flow Rate Measurements in Healthy Men and Women 20 to 30 Years of Age**

MEASUREMENT	MEN	WOMEN
FEV_T		
$\quad FEV_{0.5}$		
$\quad FEV_{1.0}$		
$\quad FEV_{2.0}$		
$\quad FEV_{3.0}$		
$FEF_{200-1200}$		
$FEF_{25\%-75\%}$		
PEFR		
MVV		

EFFECTS OF DYNAMIC COMPRESSION ON EXPIRATORY FLOW RATES

1. During approximately the first 30 percent of a forced vital capacity (FVC) maneuver, the maximum

   peak flow rate is _____

   _____

2. The first portion of the FVC (first 30%) maneuver originates from the large airways and is referred

   to as _____ .

3. Approximately the last 70 percent of a forced vital capacity maneuver is **effort independent**. Effort independent means that

   _____

   _____

   _____

4. The limitation of the flow rate that occurs during the last 70 percent of a forced vital capacity maneuver is caused by the _____ of the walls of the airway.

5. As muscular effort and intrapleural pressure increase during a forced expiratory maneuver, the **equal pressure point** moves _____ .

6. Once dynamic compression occurs during a forced expiratory maneuver, increased muscular effort (_____ increases; _____ decreases; _____ has no effect on) airway compression.

CHAPTER FIVE

THE ANATOMY AND PHYSIOLOGY OF THE CIRCULATORY SYSTEM

THE BLOOD

1. List the four major components of blood:

   a. _____

   b. _____

   c. _____

   d. _____

2. The _____ constitute the major portion of the blood cells.

3. In the healthy adult male, there are about _____ million red blood cells in each cubic millimeter of blood.

4. In the healthy adult female, there are about _____ million red blood cells in each cubic millimeter of blood.

5. The percentage of red blood cells in relation to the total blood volume is known as the

   _____ .

6. Compare the normal **hematocrit** levels for the following:

   a. Adult male _____ percent

   b. Adult female _____ percent

   c. Newborn _____ to _____ percent

7. Microscopically, the red blood cells appear as biconcave disks, averaging about _____

   in diameter and _____ in thickness.

8. The life span of an RBC is about _____ days.

9. The major function of the **leukocytes** is to _____

   _____

   _____

   _____

   _____

10. The normal amount of leukocytes averages between _____ and _____
    cells per cubic millimeter of blood.

11. Compare the normal differential count for the following:

TABLE 5–1   Normal Differential Count

POLYMORPHONUCLEAR GRANULOCYTES	MONONUCLEAR CELLS
Neutrophils	Lymphocytes
Eosinophils	Monocytes
Basophils	

12. The most numerous of the white blood cells are the _____

    _____ .

13. _____ are commonly elevated in response to an allergic condition.

14. The _____ play an important role in immunity.

15. _____ are commonly elevated in response to a chronic infection.

16. Thrombocytes are also called _____ .

17. The normal platelet count in each cubic millimeter of blood ranges between _____

    and _____ .

18. The function of the platelets is to _____

    _____

    _____

    _____

19. Plasma constitutes about _____ percent of the total blood volume.

20. Approximately _____ percent of the plasma consists of water.

21. List the three types of proteins found in the plasma:

    a. _____

    b. _____

    c. _____

22. List the electrolyte cations found in the plasma:

    a. _____

    b. _____

    c. _____

    d. _____

23. List the electrolyte anions found in the plasma:

    a. _____

    b. _____

    c. _____

    d. _____

24. List the four types of food substances found in the plasma:

    a. _____

    b. _____

    c. _____

    d. _____

25. List the four types of waste products found in the plasma:

    a. _____

    b. _____

    c. _____

    d. _____

THE HEART

1. Label and color the following anatomic structures of the heart:

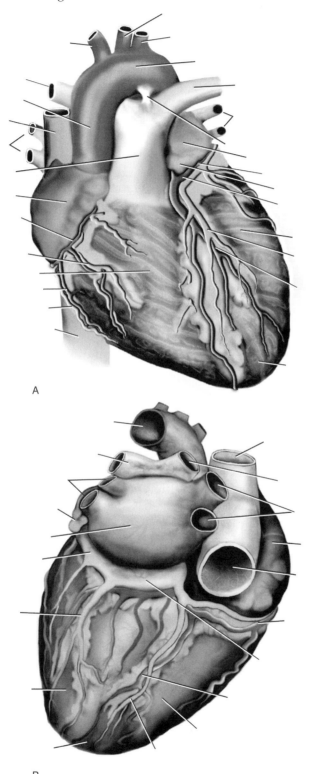

A

B

Figure 5–1   *A. Anterior view of the heart. B. Posterior view of the heart.*

2. The **heart** is a hollow, four-chambered, muscular organ that continually propels oxygen and nutrients, and consists of the upper right and left _____ and the lower right and left _____ .

3. The **atria** are separated by a thin muscular wall called the _____; the ventricles are separated by a thick muscular wall called the _____ .

4. The right atrium and ventricle act as one pump to propel _____ .

5. The left atrium and ventricle act as another pump to propel _____ .

6. The heart weighs between _____ and _____ grams.

7. When fingers are pressed between the fifth and sixth ribs just below the left nipple, the heartbeat can be felt where the apex is in contact with the internal portion of the chest. Clinically, this site is called the _____ .

The Pericardium

1. The heart is enclosed in a double-walled sac called the _____ .

2. The primary function of the **fibrous pericardium** is to

   a. _____

   b. _____

   c. _____

3. The inner wall, called the **serous pericardium**, is composed of two layers: the _____ _____ and the _____ .

The Wall of the Heart

1. The **epicardium**, or visceral layer of the pericardium, is composed of _____ _____ .

2. The **myocardium** consists of _____ _____ .

3. The **endocardium** is located in the _____ _____ .

Blood Supply of the Heart

1. The blood supply that nourishes the heart originates directly from the aorta by means of two

   arteries: the _____ and

   _____ .

2. The **left coronary artery** divides into the _____ and

   _____ .

3. The **right coronary artery** supplies the right atrium and then divides into the _____

   _____ and _____

   _____ .

4. Venous blood from the anterior side of the heart empties into the _____

   _____ .

5. Venous blood from the posterior position of the heart is collected by the _____

   _____ .

6. The **great** and **middle cardiac veins** merge and empty into a large venous cavity within the poste-

   rior wall of the right atrium called the _____ .

7. A small amount of venous blood is collected by the _____ ,
   which empties directly into both the right and left atrium.

Blood Flow through the Heart

1. The right atrium receives venous blood from the _____ and

   _____ .

2. A small amount of cardiac venous blood enters the right atrium by means of the

   _____ .

3. A one-way valve called the _____ lies between the right
   atrium and the right ventricle.

4. The tricuspid leaflets are held in place by tendinous cords called _____ .

5. The chordae tendineae are secured to the ventricular wall by the _____

   _____ .

6. When the ventricles contract, the tricuspid valve closes and blood leaves the right ventricle through

   the _____ and enters the lungs by way of the right

   and left _____ .

7. The _____ separates the right ventricle from the
   pulmonary trunk.

8. After blood passes through the lungs, it returns to the left atrium by way of the _____

   _____ .

9. The _____ lies between the left atrium and the left
   ventricle.

10. The left ventricle pumps blood through the ascending _____ .

THE PULMONARY AND SYSTEMIC VASCULAR SYSTEMS

1. The **pulmonary circulation system** begins with the _____ and

   ends in the _____ .

2. The **systemic circulation system** begins with the _____ and ends

   in the _____ .

3. The **arteries** are vessels that carry blood (_____ to; _____ away from) the heart.

4. The arteries subdivide into smaller vessels called _____ .

5. The _____ play a major role in the distribution and regulation of blood pressure.

6. Which vessels are referred to as the **resistance vessels**?

   Answer: _____ .

7. In the **capillaries** of the pulmonary system, gas exchange is called _____ respiration.

8. In the capillaries of the systemic system, gas exchange is called _____ respiration.

9. Tiny vessels continuous with the capillaries are called _____ .

10. Veins are also known as _____ vessels.

11. Approximately _____ percent of the body's total blood volume is contained within the venous system.

12. The pulmonary **arterioles** and most of the arterioles in the systemic circulation are controlled by

   _____ impulses.

13. The _____ center, located in the _____ , governs

   the number of _____ impulses sent to the vascular systems.

14. Under normal circumstances, a continual stream of _____ impulses are sent to blood vessels.

15. A moderate state of constant vascular constriction is called _____ .

16. When the **vasomotor center** is activated to constrict a particular vascular region, it does so by

   (_____ increasing; _____ decreasing) the number of _____ impulses sent to that vascular area.

17. When the vasomotor center causes vasodilation, it does so by (_____ increasing; _____ decreasing)

   the number of _____ impulses sent to that vascular region.

18. List the major vascular beds in the systemic system that dilate in response to sympathetic impulses:

    The arterioles of the

    a. _____

    b. _____

    c. _____

19. **Baroreceptors**, which are specialized stretch receptors, are also called _____

    _____ .

20. The baroreceptors located in the **carotid arteries** send neural impulses to the medulla by means of

    the _____ nerve.

21. The baroreceptors located in the arch of the aorta send neural impulses to the medulla by means of

    the _____ nerve.

22. When the arterial blood pressure decreases, neural impulses to the medulla (_____ increase; _____

    decrease), which, in turn, causes the medulla to (_____ increase; _____ decrease) its sympathetic
    activity.

23. When the baroreceptors signal the medulla to increase its sympathetic activity, the net result is

    a. _____

    _____

    b. _____

    _____

    c. _____

    _____

24. In addition to the baroreceptors located in the carotid sinuses and aortic arch, other baroreceptors
    are found in the

    a. _____

    b. _____

    c. _____

    d. _____

PRESSURES IN THE PULMONARY AND SYSTEMIC VASCULAR SYSTEMS

1. **Intravascular pressure** is defined as the _____

_____

_____

_____

2. **Transmural pressure** is defined as the _____

_____

_____

_____

_____

3. A positive transmural pressure is when pressure inside the vessel is (_____ greater than; _____ less than; _____ the same as) the pressure outside the vessel.

4. A negative transmural pressure is when the pressure inside the vessel is (_____ greater than; _____ less than; _____ the same as) the pressure outside the vessel.

5. **Driving pressure** is defined as the _____

_____

_____

_____

THE CARDIAC CYCLE AND ITS EFFECT ON BLOOD PRESSURE

1. The maximum pressure generated during ventricular contraction is the _____ .

2. When the ventricles relax, the lowest pressure that remains in the arteries prior to the next ventricular contraction is the _____ .

3. What is the MAP in an individual who has a systolic pressure of 165 mm Hg and a diastolic pressure of 105 mm Hg?

Answer: _____

4. Compared to the pulmonary circulation, the minimum pressure in the systemic system is about

    _____ times greater.

5. Using the illustration below, identify the mean intraluminal blood pressures at the points indicated in the pulmonary and systemic circulation:

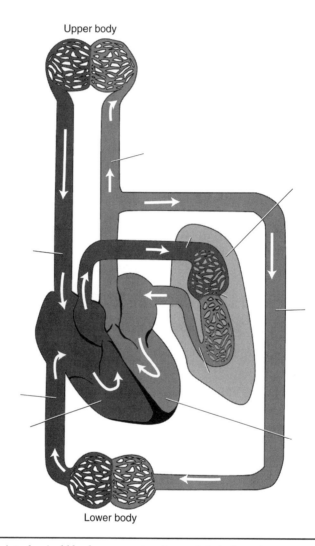

Figure 5–2 *Mean intraluminal blood pressure at various points in the pulmonary and systemic circulation.*

6. Normally, the **stroke volume** ranges between _____ and _____ .

7. The total volume of blood discharged from the ventricles per minute is called _____

    _____ .

8. If an individual has a stroke volume of 55 mL, and a heart rate of 80 beats per minute (beats/min), what is the cardiac output?

   Answer: _____

9. Under normal conditions, when either the stroke volume or heart rate increases, the blood pressure

   a. increases
   b. decreases
   c. remains the same

10. The normal adult total blood volume is about _____ liters.

11. In regard to the total blood volume of the normal adults, about _____ percent is in the systemic

    circulation, _____ percent is in the heart, and _____ percent is in the pulmonary circulation.

12. Overall, about _____ percent of the total blood volume is in the veins, and about _____ percent is in the arteries.

THE DISTRIBUTION OF PULMONARY BLOOD FLOW

1. The fact that blood is **gravity dependent** means that it naturally moves _____

   _____

   _____

   _____

2. The intraluminal pressures in the vessels of the gravity-dependent area of the lung are (_____

   greater than; _____ less than; _____ the same as) the intraluminal pressures in the least gravity-dependent area.

3. When an individual is in each of the following positions, which part of the lung is the gravity-dependent region?

BODY POSITION	GRAVITY-DEPENDENT LUNG REGION
a. Lying on the back	_____
b. Lying on the stomach	_____
c. Lying on the side	_____
d. Suspended upside down	_____

4. In **Zone 1** of the upright lung, the alveolar pressure is sometimes (_____ greater than; _____ less than; _____ the same as) both the arterial and the venous intraluminal pressures.

5. List some conditions that can cause the alveolar pressure to be higher than the arterial and venous pressures:

   a. _____

   b. _____

   c. _____

6. When the alveoli are ventilated but not perfused, _____ is said to exist.

7. In **Zone 2** of the upright lung, the arterial intraluminal pressure is (_____ greater than; _____ less than; _____ the same as) the alveolar pressure; and the alveolar pressure is (_____ greater than; _____ less than; _____ the same as) the venous pressure.

8. In **Zone 3** of the upright lung, the arterial intraluminal pressure is (_____ greater than; _____ less than; _____ the same as) the alveolar pressure; and the alveolar pressure is (_____ greater than; _____ less than; _____ the same as) the venous pressure.

9. List the three mechanisms that determine stroke volume:

   a. _____

   b. _____

   c. _____

10. **Ventricular preload** refers to _____

    _____

    _____

11. Within limits, the more myocardial fiber is stretched during diastole, the (_____ more; _____ less) strongly it will contract during systole.

12. **VEDP** stands for _____ .

13. **VEDV** stands for _____ .

14. As the VEDV increases the VEDP

    a. increases
    b. decreases
    c. remains the same

15. The relationship between the VEDP and cardiac output is known as the _____

    _____ .

16. **Ventricular afterload** is defined as _____

    _____

    _____

17. Ventricular afterload is determined by

    a. _____

    _____

    b. _____

    _____

    c. _____

    _____

18. Clinically, what reflects the ventricular afterload the best?

    Answer: _____

19. Blood pressure (BP) equals

    BP = _____ × _____

20. **Myocardial contractility** can be pictured as _____

    _____

    _____

    _____

21. In general, when the contractility of the heart decreases, the cardiac output
    a. increases
    b. decreases
    c. remains the same

22. List some clinical assessments that reflect myocardial contractility.

    a. _____

    b. _____

    c. _____

    d. _____

23. An increase in myocardial contractility is referred to as _____

    _____.

24. A decrease in myocardial contractility is referred to as _____

    _____.

25. Circulatory resistance is derived as follows:

    Resistance =

26. In general, when the vascular resistance increases, the blood pressure
    a. increases
    b. decreases
    c. remains the same

Active Mechanisms Affecting Vascular Resistance

1. Define **active mechanism**: _____

   _____

   _____

   _____

2. In response to a decreased alveolar oxygen pressure, the pulmonary vascular system

   a. constricts
   b. relaxes
   c. remains the same

3. In response to an increased P_{CO_2} level, the pulmonary vascular system

   a. constricts
   b. relaxes
   c. remains the same

4. In response to a decreased pH, the pulmonary vascular system

   a. constricts
   b. relaxes
   c. remains the same

5. In response to an increased H^+ concentration, the pulmonary vascular system

   a. constricts
   b. relaxes
   c. remains the same

6. List some pharmacologic agents that constrict the pulmonary vessels:

   a. _____

   b. _____

   c. _____

   d. _____

   e. _____

7. List some pharmacologic agents that relax the pulmonary vessels:

a. _____

b. _____

c. _____

d. _____

8. List some pathologic conditions that increase pulmonary vascular resistance:

a. _____

b. _____

c. _____

d. _____

Passive Mechanisms Affecting Vascular Resistance

1. Define **passive mechanism**: _____

_____

_____

_____

2. In response to an increased pulmonary arterial pressure, the pulmonary vascular resistance
   a. increases
   b. decreases
   c. remains the same

3. The answer to the above question occurs because of **recruitment**, which entails _____

_____

_____

and because of distention, which entails _____

_____

_____

4. In response to an increased left atrial pressure, the pulmonary vascular resistance

   a. increases
   b. decreases
   c. remains the same

5. At high lung volumes, the pulmonary resistance in the **alveolar vessels** is (_____ high; _____ low).

6. At high lung volumes, the pulmonary resistance in the **extra-alveolar vessels** is (_____ high;

   _____ low).

7. At low lung volumes, the pulmonary resistance in the alveolar vessels is (_____ high; _____ low).

8. At low lung volumes, the pulmonary resistance in the extra-alveolar vessels is (_____ high;

   _____ low).

9. At high lung volumes, the pulmonary vascular resistance in the corner vessels is (_____ high;

   _____ low).

10. At low lung volumes, the pulmonary vascular resistance in the corner vessels is (_____ high;

    _____ low).

11. In response to an increased blood volume, pulmonary vascular resistance

    a. increases
    b. decreases
    c. remains the same

12. In response to an increased blood viscosity, the pulmonary vascular resistance

    a. increases
    b. decreases
    c. remains the same

CHAPTER SIX

OXYGEN TRANSPORT

OXYGEN TRANSPORT

1. Compare the normal ranges for the following blood gas values:

TABLE 6–1 **Normal Blood Gas Value Ranges**

BLOOD GAS VALUE	ARTERIAL	VENOUS
pH		
P_{CO_2}		
HCO_3^-		
P_{O_2}		

2. The term **dissolve** means that when a gas like oxygen enters the plasma, it _____

_____

_____

3. Clinically, which portion of the oxygen transport system is measured to assess the patient's partial pressure of oxygen (P_{O_2})?

Answer: _____

4. Complete the following exercise:

   a. If an individual has an arterial oxygen partial pressure (Pa_{O_2}) of 50 mm Hg, about how many mL of oxygen are dissolved in every 100 mL of blood?

   Answer: _____ mL O_2/100 mL of blood

   b. In regard to the above answer, what is the vol% of dissolved oxygen?

   Answer: _____

5. Vol% (volume percent) is defined as _____

   _____

6. Each red blood cell (RBC) contains approximately _____ million hemoglobin molecules.

7. The normal adult hemoglobin is designated as Hb _____.

8. In the normal adult hemoglobin, how many heme group(s) are there?

   Answer: _____

9. Write the reversible reaction of O_2 with Hb:

10. When two oxygen molecules are bound to one Hb molecule, the Hb is said to be _____ percent saturated with oxygen; an Hb molecule with one oxygen molecule is _____ percent saturated.

11. Hemoglobin bound with oxygen is called _____ .

12. Hemoglobin not bound with oxygen is called _____

    or _____ .

13. The amount of oxygen bound to hemoglobin is (_____ indirectly; _____ directly) related to the partial pressure of oxygen.

14. The globin portion of each hemoglobin molecule consists of _____

    _____

    _____

    _____

15. Fetal hemoglobin (HbF) has _____ chains and _____ chains.

16. Hemoglobin changed from the ferrous state to the ferric state is known as _____

    _____ .

17. Compare the normal hemoglobin values for the following:

    a. Adult male: _____ g% Hb

    b. Adult female: _____ g% Hb

    c. Average infant: _____ g% Hb

18. Hemoglobin constitutes about _____ percent of the RBC weight.

19. Each gram percent (g%) Hb is capable of carrying about _____ mL of oxygen.

20. At a normal arterial oxygen pressure (Pa_{O_2}) the hemoglobin saturation (Sa_{O_2}) is only 97 percent because of the following normal physiologic shunts:

    a. _____

    _____

    b. _____

    _____

    c. _____

    _____

21. Complete the following total oxygen transport exercises:

Case A

A 23-year-old female with severe asthma presents with the following clinical data:

Hb: 13 g%
Pa_{O_2}: 55 mm Hg
Sa_{O_2}: 85%
Cardiac output: 6 L/min

a. How much dissolved O_2 is the patient transporting in every 100 mL of blood?

Answer: _____ mL O_2/100 mL blood (vol%)

b. How much O_2 is bound to the hemoglobin in every 100 mL of blood?

Answer: _____ mL O_2/100 mL blood (vol%)

c. What is the total O_2 content of the arterial blood (Ca_{O_2})?

Answer: Ca_{O_2} = _____ (vol% O_2 or mL O_2/100 mL blood)

d. As the Ca_{O_2} is in reference to 1/10 of 1 liter of blood, how many mL of O_2 are available for tissue metabolism in one liter of blood?

Answer: _____ mL O_2/liter

e. As this patient has a cardiac output of 6 L/min, how many mL of O_2 are available for tissue metabolism in 1 minute?

Answer: _____ mL O_2/min

Case B

A 62-year-old male with severe emphysema presents with the following clinical data:

- Hb: 18 g%
- Pa_{O_2}: 50 mm Hg
- Sa_{O_2}: 80%
- Cardiac output: 3.5 L/min
- $P\bar{v}_{O_2}$: 25 mm Hg
- $S\bar{v}_{O_2}$: 50%
- PA_{O_2}: 150 mm Hg

a. How much dissolved O_2 is the patient transporting in every 100 mL of blood?

Answer: _____ mL O_2/100 mL blood (vol%)

b. How much O_2 is bound to the hemoglobin in every 100 mL of blood?

Answer: _____ mL O_2/100 mL blood (vol% O_2)

c. What is the total O_2 content of the arterial blood (Ca_{O_2})?

Answer: Ca_{O_2} = _____ (vol% O_2 or mL O_2/100 mL blood)

d. As the Ca_{O_2} is in reference to 1/10 of 1 liter of blood, how many mL of O_2 are available for tissue metabolism in 1 liter of blood?

Answer: _____ mL O_2/liter

e. As this patient has a cardiac output of 3.5 L/min, how many mL of O_2 are available for tissue metabolism in 1 minute?

Answer: _____ mL O_2/min

f. What is the patient's total oxygen content of mixed venous blood ($C\bar{v}_{O_2}$)?

Answer: $C\bar{v}_{O_2}$ = _____ (vol% O_2 or mL O_2/100 mL blood)

g. What is the patient's total oxygen content of capillary blood (Cc_{O_2})?

Answer: Cc_{O_2} = _____ (vol% O_2 or mL O_2/100 mL blood)

OXYGEN DISSOCIATION CURVE

1. The **oxygen dissociation curve** illustrates the _____ of hemoglobin that is

   chemically bound to oxygen at each oxygen _____ .

2. Clinically, the flat portion of the oxygen dissociation curve is significant because it illustrates that

   a. _____

   _____

   b. _____

   _____

   c. _____

   _____

3. Clinically, the steep portion of the oxygen dissociation curve is significant because it illustrates that

   a. _____

   _____

   _____

   b. _____

   _____

4. Using the oxygen dissociation curve nomogram below, answer the next two questions (a and b).

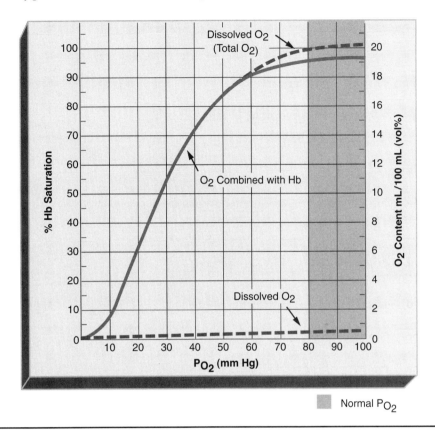

Figure 6–1 *Oxygen dissociation curve.*

a. If the P_{O_2} is 50 mm Hg, what is the percentage of hemoglobin that is bound to oxygen?

Answer: _____

b. What is the oxygen content level in vol%?

Answer: _____

5. The **P$_{50}$** represents _____

6. Normally, the P_{50} is about _____ mm Hg.

7. When the oxygen dissociation curve shifts to the right, the P_{50}

    a. increases
    b. decreases
    c. remains the same

8. When the oxygen dissociation curve shifts to the left, the P_{50}

    a. increases
    b. decreases
    c. remains the same

9. List factors that shift the oxygen dissociation curve to the

    a. left: _____

       _____

       _____

       _____

       _____

       _____

    b. right: _____

       _____

       _____

       _____

10. Clinically, when the oxygen dissociation curve shifts to the *right*, the loading of oxygen in the lungs at any given P_{O_2}

    a. increases
    b. decreases
    c. remains the same

11. Clinically, when the oxygen dissociation curve shifts to the *right*, the plasma P_{O_2} reduction necessary to unload oxygen at the tissue sites is

    a. less than normal
    b. greater than normal
    c. the same as normal

12. Clinically, when the oxygen dissociation curve shifts to the *left*, the loading of oxygen in the lungs at any given P_{O_2}

    a. increases
    b. decreases
    c. remains the same

13. Clinically, when the oxygen dissociation curve shifts to the *left*, the plasma P_{O_2} reduction necessary to unload oxygen at the tissue sites is

    a. less than normal
    b. greater than normal
    c. the same as normal

OXYGEN TRANSPORT CALCULATIONS

1. List the most common oxygen transport studies performed in the clinical setting:

    a. _____

    b. _____

    c. _____

    d. _____

    e. _____

    f. _____

2. **Total oxygen delivery** to the peripheral tissues is dependent on the

    a. _____

    b. _____

    c. _____

3. Complete the following formula:

    $D_{O_2} =$

4. If a patient has a cardiac output of 3.5 L/min and a Ca_{O_2} of 12 vol%, what is the total amount of oxygen delivered to the patient's peripheral cells?

Answer: _____

5. List three conditions that reduce an individual's total oxygen delivery:

a. _____

b. _____

c. _____

6. The **arterial-venous content difference** $[C(a - v)_{O_2}]$ is defined as the difference _____

_____

_____

7. Complete the following formula:

$$C(a - \bar{v})_{O_2} =$$

8. If a patient has a Ca_{O_2} of 13 vol% and a $C\bar{v}_{O_2}$ of 9 vol%, what is the patient's $C(a - \bar{v})_{O_2}$?

Answer: _____

9. List some clinical factors that *increase* the $C(a - \bar{v})_{O_2}$:

a. _____

b. _____

1. _____

2. _____

3. _____

4. _____

10. List some clinical factors that *decrease* the $C(a - \bar{v})_{O_2}$:

    a. _____

    b. _____

    c. _____

    d. _____

    e. _____

11. The amount of oxygen extracted by the peripheral tissues during the period of 1 minute is called

    _____ or _____ .

12. Complete the following formula:

    $$\dot{V}_{O_2} =$$

13. If a patient has a cardiac output of 7.5 L/min and a $C(a - \bar{v})_{O_2}$ of 8 vol%, what is the patient's $\dot{V}_{O_2}$?

    Answer: _____

14. List some clinical factors that *increase* the $\dot{V}_{O_2}$:

    a. _____

    b. _____

    c. _____

    d. _____

15. List some clinical factors that *decrease* the $\dot{V}_{O_2}$:

    a. _____

    b. _____

    c. _____

    d. _____

16. An individual's oxygen consumption index is derived by dividing the $\dot{V}_{O_2}$ by the _____

   _____.

17. The average oxygen consumption index ranges between _____ and _____ $mL\,O_2/m^2$.

18. The oxygen extraction ratio (O_2ER) is defined as the amount of oxygen _____

   _____

   _____

   _____

   _____

19. The O_2ER is also known as the

   a. _____

   b. _____

20. Complete the following formula:

   $O_2ER =$

21. The normal O_2ER is _____ percent.

22. a. If a patient has a Ca_{O_2} of 14 vol%, and a $C\bar{v}_{O_2}$ of 7 vol%, what is the patient's O_2ER?

   Answer: _____ percent

   b. If the above patient has a total oxygen delivery of 850 mL/minute, then this would mean that

   during a course of 1 minute, _____ mL of oxygen are metabolized by the tissues and

   _____ mL of oxygen are returned to the lungs.

23. List some clinical factors that *increase* the O_2ER:

    a. _____

    b. _____

        1. _____

        2. _____

        3. _____

        4. _____

    c. _____

    d. _____

24. List some clinical factors that *decrease* the O_2ER:

    a. _____

    b. _____

    c. _____

    d. _____

    e. _____

    f. _____

    g. _____

25. The normal $S\bar{v}_{O_2}$ is _____ percent.

26. Clinically, an $S\bar{v}_{O_2}$ of about _____ percent is acceptable.

27. List some clinical factors that *decrease* the $S\bar{v}_{O_2}$:

a. _____

b. _____

1. _____

2. _____

3. _____

4. _____

28. A reduction in the $S\bar{v}_{O_2}$ indicates that the $C(a - \bar{v})_{O_2}$, $\dot{V}_{O_2}$, and O_2ER are

a. increasing
b. decreasing
c. remaining the same

29. List some clinical factors that *increase* the $S\bar{v}_{O_2}$:

a. _____

b. _____

c. _____

d. _____

e. _____

30. An increase in the $S\bar{v}_{O_2}$ indicates that the $C(a - \bar{v})_{O_2}$, $\dot{V}_{O_2}$, and O_2ER are

a. increasing
b. decreasing
c. remaining the same

31. Fill in the blanks under each major sub-heading shown in the Clinical Factors column. Also, fill in the blanks provided under the Oxygen Transport Calculations; use the following code: Same = unchanged status; ↑ = increase; ↓ = decrease.

TABLE 6–2 Clinical Factors Affecting Various Oxygen Transport Calculation Values

| CLINICAL FACTORS | OXYGEN TRANSPORT CALCULATION | | | | |
	D_{O_2} (1000 mL O_2/min)	$\dot{V}_{O_2}$ (250 mL O_2/min)	$C(a-\bar{v})_{O_2}$ (5 vol%)	O_2ER (25%)	$S\bar{v}_{O_2}$ (75%)
↑ O_2 Loading in the lungs	____	____	____	____	____
_____					
_____					
_____					
_____					
↓ O_2 Loading in the lungs	____	____	____	____	____
_____					
_____					
_____					
_____					
_____					
↑ Metabolism	____	____	____	____	____
_____					
_____					
_____					
↓ Metabolism	____	____	____	____	____
_____					
↑ Cardiac output	____	____	____	____	____
↓ Cardiac output	____	____	____	____	____
Peripheral shunting	____	____	____	____	____
Certain poisons	____	____	____	____	____

PULMONARY SHUNTING

1. **Pulmonary shunting** is defined as _____

   _____

   _____

   _____

   _____

   _____

   _____

2. **Absolute shunts** (true shunts) can be grouped under the following two categories:

   a. _____

   b. _____

3. An **anatomic shunt** exists when _____

   _____

   _____

   _____

4. In the healthy lung, the normal anatomic shunt is about _____ percent.

5. List three common causes of **anatomic shunting**.

   a. _____

   b. _____

   c. _____

6. List three common causes of **capillary shunts**.

   a. _____

   b. _____

   c. _____

7. The sum of the anatomic and capillary shunts is referred to as the _____ or

   _____ .

8. What does refractory to oxygen therapy mean? _____

_____

_____

_____

_____

_____

9. A **relative shunt** or **shunt-like effect** is said to exist when _____

_____

_____

10. List three common causes of a relative shunt or shunt-like effect.

    a. _____

    b. _____

    c. _____

11. What is **venous admixture**? _____

_____

_____

_____

12. Complete the following shunt equation:

$$\frac{\dot{Q}s}{\dot{Q}T} =$$

13. A 42-year-old female is on a volume-cycled mechanical ventilator on a day when the barometric pressure is 740 mm Hg. The patient is receiving an $F_{I_{O_2}}$ of 0.45. The following clinical data are obtained:

Hb: 10 g%

Pa_{O_2}: 65 mm Hg (Sa_{O_2} = 91%)

Pa_{CO_2}: 35 mm Hg

$P\bar{v}_{O_2}$: 30 mm Hg ($S\bar{v}_{O_2}$ = 60%)

Using the information above, calculate the patient's $P_{A_{O_2}}$, Cc_{O_2}, Ca_{O_2}, and $C\bar{v}_{O_2}$.

a. $P_{A_{O_2}}$ =

Answer: _____

b. Cc_{O_2} =

Answer: _____

c. Ca_{O_2} =

Answer: _____

d. $C\bar{v}_{O_2}$ =

Answer: _____

e. Using the clinical data above, calculate the patient's pulmonary shunt:

$$\frac{\dot{Q}s}{\dot{Q}T} =$$

Answer: _____

14. What is the clinical significance of the following calculated shunts:

a. below 10 percent: _____

_____

b. 10–20 percent: _____

_____

c. 20–30 percent: _____

_____

d. greater than 30 percent: _____

_____

15. List three clinical factors that cause the calculation of pulmonary shunting to be unreliable:

a. _____

b. _____

c. _____

HYPOXEMIA VERSUS HYPOXIA

1. **Hypoxemia** refers to _____

_____

_____

2. What are the Pa_{O_2} ranges for the following hypoxemia classifications?

   a. Mild hypoxemia   _____

   b. Moderate hypoxemia   _____

   c. Severe hypoxemia   _____

3. **Hypoxia** refers to _____

4. List four common causes of **hypoxic hypoxia**.

   a. _____

   b. _____

   c. _____

   d. _____

5. **Anemic hypoxia** is described as occurring when _____

_____

_____

_____

_____

6. Anemic hypoxia can develop from

   a. _____

   b. _____

7. **Circulatory hypoxia** is defined as occurring when _____

_____

_____

_____

8. The two main causes of circulator hypoxia are

a. _____

b. _____

9. **Histotoxic hypoxia** is defined as _____

_____

_____

10. Define **cyanosis**: _____

_____

_____

11. Define **polycythemia**: _____

_____

_____

CHAPTER SEVEN

CARBON DIOXIDE TRANSPORT AND ACID-BASE BALANCE

CARBON DIOXIDE TRANSPORT

1. List the three ways that carbon dioxide is transported from the tissue cells to the lungs in the **plasma**:

   a. _____

   b. _____

   c. _____

2. List the three ways that carbon dioxide is transported from the tissue cells to the lungs in the **red blood cells**:

   a. _____

   b. _____

   c. _____

3. In what form is most of the carbon dioxide carried to the lungs?

   Answer: _____

4. The answer to the above question accounts for about _____ percent of the total amount of carbon dioxide transported to the lungs.

5. Using the following illustration, write the various chemical reaction(s) carbon dioxide goes through at the tissue sites to be transported to the lungs.

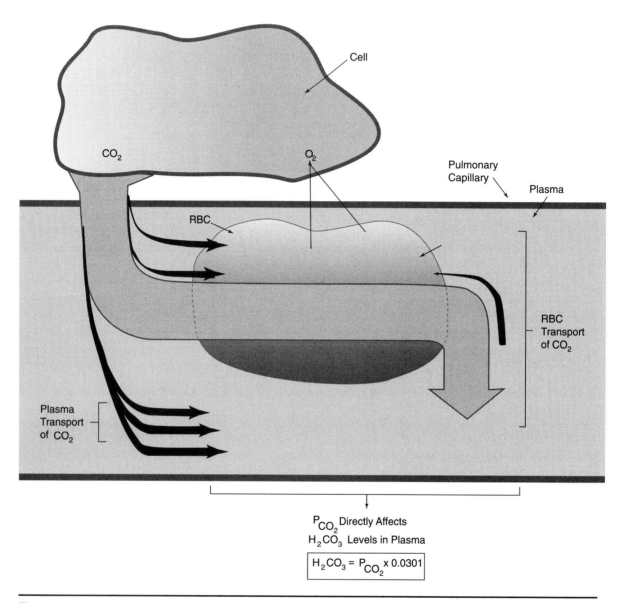

$$H_2CO_3 = P_{CO_2} \times 0.0301$$

Figure 7–1   *How CO_2 is converted to HCO_3^- at the tissue sites. Most of the CO_2 that is produced at the tissue cells is carried to the lungs in the form of HCO_3^-.*

CARBON DIOXIDE DISSOCIATION CURVE

1. Unlike the S-shaped oxygen dissociation curve, the carbon dioxide curve is much more

   _____ .

2. Using the following carbon dioxide dissociation curve nomogram, if the P_{CO_2} increases from 25 mm Hg

   to 40 mm Hg, the carbon dioxide content increases from _____ vol% to _____ vol%.

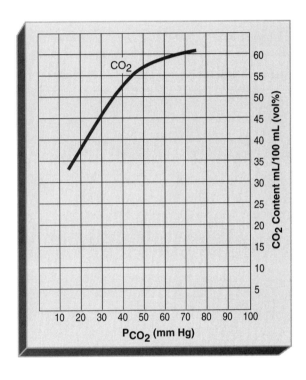

3. The fact that deoxygenated blood enhances the loading of carbon dioxide is called the

   _____ .

ACID-BASE BALANCE AND REGULATION

1. The normal arterial pH range is _____ to _____ .

2. The normal venous pH range is _____ to _____ .

3. When the pH of the arterial blood is greater than 7.45, _____ or _____ is said to exist.

4. When the pH falls below 7.35, _____ or _____ is said to be present.

5. Most H$^+$ ions in the body originate from

   a. _____

   b. _____

   c. _____

   d. _____

6. Under normal conditions, both the H$^+$ and HCO$_3^-$ ion concentrations in the blood are regulated by the following three major systems:

   a. _____

   b. _____

   c. _____

7. The **chemical buffer system** responds within a fraction of a second to resist pH changes, and is called the _____.

8. The chemical buffer system inactivates _____ and liberates _____ in response to acidosis, or generate more H$^+$ ions and decreases the concentration of HCO$_3^-$ ions in response to _____.

9. The respiratory system acts within ____ to ____ minutes by increasing or decreasing the breathing _____ and _____ to offset acidosis or alkalosis, respectively.

10. The renal system is the body's _____.

11. The renal system requires a _____ to correct abnormal pH concentrations.

12. When the extracellular fluids become acidic, the renal system retains _____ and excretes _____ ions into the urine, causing the blood pH to _____.

13. On the other hand, when the extracellular fluids become alkaline, the renal system _____ _____ and _____ into the urine, causing the blood pH to _____.

The Basic Principles of Acid-Base Reactions and pH

Acids and Bases

1. Similar to salts, _____. Thus, both acids and bases can

    a. _____

    b. _____

Acids

1. An **acid** is a substance that _____ in measurable amounts.

2. Acids are defined as _____.

3. The acidity of a solution reflects only the _____, not those bound to anions.

4. Hydrochloric acid (HCl), the acid found in the stomach that works to aid digestion, dissociates into a proton and a chloride ion. Write the equation in the space provided below.

Strong and Weak Acids

1. The acidity of a solution reflects only the _____—not the _____.

2. **Strong acids** dissociate _____ (i.e., _____) and _____ in water.

3. If 100 hydrochloric (HCl) acid molecules were placed in 1 mL of water, the hydrochloric acid would

    dissociate into _____ and _____ ions.

4. **Weak acids** do _____ in a solution.

5. Examples of weak acids are _____ and _____.

6. If 100 acetic acid molecules were placed in 1 mL of water, the following reaction would occur (write the equation in the space provided below):

    $100 \ HC_2H_3O_2$

Bases

1. **Bases** are _____.

2. A base is a substance that _____ in measurable amounts.

3. Similar to acids, when dissolved in water, hydroxides dissociate into _____.

4. Ionization of sodium hydroxide (NaOH) results in a hydroxide ion and a sodium ion. The liberated hydroxide ion then bonds, or accepts, a proton present in the solution. This reaction produces water and, at the same time, decreases the acidity [H^+ concentration] of the solution. Write this equation in the space provided below.

5. The _____ is an important base in the body and is especially abundant in the blood.

6. _____, a natural waste product of protein breakdown, is also a base. _____ has a pair of unshared electrons that strongly attract protons.

Strong and Weak Bases

1. Bases are _____ .

2. **Strong bases** (e.g., hydroxides) dissociate easily in water and quickly tie up _____.

3. **Weak bases** (e.g., sodium bicarbonate or baking soda) _____ and _____ and are

   _____.

4. Because sodium bicarbonate accepts a relatively small amount of protons, its released bicarbonate

   ion is described _____.

pH: Acid-Base Concentration

1. As the concentration of _____ in a solution increases, the more acidic the solution becomes.

2. On the other hand, as the level of _____ increases, the more basic, or alkaline, the solution becomes.

3. Clinically, the concentration of hydrogen ions in the body is measured in units called _____.

4. The pH scale runs from _____ and is _____.

5. Each successive unit change in pH represents a _____ change in hydrogen ion concentration.

6. The pH of a solution is defined as _____

_____:

pH =

7. When the pH is 7 ($H^+ = 10^{-7}$ mol/L), the number of _____,

and the solution is neutral—that is, neither _____ nor _____.

8. Pure water has a neutral pH of _____ or _____ ions.

9. A solution with a pH below 7 is _____—that is, there are _____ ions.

10. A solution with a pH of 6 has _____ ions than a solution with a pH of _____.

11. A solution with a pH greater than 7 is _____—that is, the _____ ions.

12. A solution with a pH of 8 has _____ ions than a solution with a pH of _____.

13. As the hydrogen ion concentration increases, the hydroxide ion concentration _____.

The Chemical Buffer Systems and Acid-Base Balance

1. Chemical buffers resist pH changes and are the body's _____.

2. The ability of an acid-base mixture to resist sudden changes in pH is called its _____.

3. Buffers work against sudden and large changes in the pH of body fluids by (1) _____

_____, and (2) _____.

4. The three major chemical buffer systems in the body are the _____.

Carbonic Acid-Bicarbonate Buffer System and Acid-Base Balance

1. The **carbonic acid-bicarbonate buffer system** plays an extremely important role in maintaining pH homeostasis of the blood. Carbonic acid (H_2CO_3) dissociates reversibly and releases bicarbonate ions (HCO_3^-) and protons (H^+) as follows (write the equation in the space provided):

H_2CO_3

2. The carbonic acid-bicarbonate buffer system converts

   a. _____

   b. _____

The Henderson-Hasselbalch Equation

1. The **Henderson-Hasselbalch equation** uses the components of the H_2CO_3/HCO_3 system in the following way (write the equation in the space provided):

   $$pH = pK$$

2. The pK is derived from _____.

3. Normally the pK is _____.

4. The normal HCO_3 to H_2CO_3 ratio is _____.

5. An HCO_3 to H_2CO_3 ratio of 17:1 means the pH is
   a. normal
   b. less than normal
   c. greater than normal

6. An HCO_3 to H_2CO_3 ratio of 26:1 means the pH is
   a. normal
   b. less than normal
   c. greater than normal

Phosphate Buffer System and Acid-Base Balance

1. The primary components of the **phosphate buffer system** are the _____ and

   _____.

2. NaH_2PO_4 is a weak _____.

3. Na_2HPO_4, which has one less hydrogen atom, is a weak _____.

4. The phosphate buffer system is only about _____ as effective as the carbonic acid-bicarbonate buffer system in the extracellular fluid.

Protein Buffer System and Acid-Base Balance

1. The **protein buffer system,** the body's most abundant and influential supply of buffers is found in

   the _____ the _____ and _____ .

2. About _____ of the buffering power of body fluids is found in the intracellular proteins.

3. Proteins are _____ of amino acids.

4. Some of the amino acids have exposed groups of atoms known as _____ ,

   which dissociate and _____ in response to _____ .

5. Other amino acids consist of exposed groups that can function as bases and _____ .

6. Protein molecules that have a reversible ability are called _____ .

7. The hemoglobin in red blood cells is a good example of a protein that works as an

   _____ .

8. CO_2 released at the tissue cells quickly forms _____ , and then dissociates into ___ and ___
   ions. At the same time, the hemoglobin is unloading oxygen at the tissue sites and becoming

   _____ .

9. True ___ False ___ Reduced hemoglobin carries a negative charge.

10. True ___ False ___ H_2CO_3 is a weaker acid than the hemoglobin protein.

The Respiratory System and Acid-Base Balance

1. Although the respiratory system does not respond as fast as the chemical buffer systems, it has up

   to _____ times the buffering power of all of the chemical buffer systems combined.

2. The CO_2 produced at the tissue cells enters the red blood cells and is converted to HCO_3^- ions as
   follows (write the equation in the space provided):

   $CO_2 +$

3. True ____ False ____ Under normal conditions, the volume of CO_2 eliminated at the lung is equal to the amount of CO_2 produced at the tissues.

4. When the pH declines (e.g., metabolic acidosis caused by lactic acids), the respiratory system

   responds by _____ the breathing depth and rate.

5. When the pH rises (e.g., metabolic alkalosis caused by hypokalemia), the respiratory system

   responds by _____ the breathing depth and rate.

6. True ____ False ____ When the volume of CO_2 expelled from the lungs is greater than the amount of CO_2 produced at the tissue cells, **hypoventilation** is present.

7. True ____ False ____ When the volume of CO_2 eliminated from the lungs is less than the amount of CO_2 produced at the tissue cells, **respiratory acidosis** is said to exist.

The Renal System and Acid-Base Balance

1. Only the renal system can rid the body of acids such as _____ , _____ ,

   _____ , and _____ .

2. Only the renal system can regulate _____ in the blood and _____ that are used up in managing the H^+ levels in the extracellular fluids.

3. When the extracellular fluids become acidic, the renal system _____ and excretes _____ ions

   into the urine, causing the blood pH to _____ .

4. When the extracellular fluids become alkaline, the renal system _____ and excretes _____

   substances into the urine, causing the blood pH to _____ .

THE ROLE OF THE P_{CO_2}/HCO_3^-/pH RELATIONSHIP IN ACID-BASE BALANCE

Acid-Base Balance Disturbances

1. Hypoventilation causes the partial pressure of the alveolar carbon dioxide ($P_{A_{CO_2}}$) to increase, which in turn causes the following plasma components to

    a. P_{CO_2} (_____ increase; _____ decrease; _____ remain the same)

    b. HCO_3^- (_____ increase; _____ decrease; _____ remain the same)

    c. H_2CO_3 (_____ increase; _____ decrease; _____ remain the same)

    d. HCO_3^- : H_2CO_3 ratio (_____ increase; _____ decrease; _____ remain the same)

    e. pH (_____ increase; _____ decrease; _____ remain the same)

2. Hyperventilation causes the partial pressure of the alveolar carbon dioxide ($P_{A_{CO_2}}$) to increase, which in turn causes the following plasma components to

    a. P_{CO_2} (_____ increase; _____ decrease; _____ remain the same)

    b. HCO_3^- (_____ increase; _____ decrease; _____ remain the same)

    c. H_2CO_3 (_____ increase; _____ decrease; _____ remain the same)

    d. HCO_3^- : H_2CO_3 ratio (_____ increase; _____ decrease; _____ remain the same)

    e. pH (_____ increase; _____ decrease; _____ remain the same)

Respiratory Acid-Base Disturbances

Acute Ventilatory Failure (Respiratory Acidosis)

1. Using the P_{CO_2}/HCO_3/pH nomogram provided below, if a patient's ventilatory rate suddenly decreased and caused the patient's $P_{A_{CO_2}}$ to increase to 70 mm Hg, what approximate changes would be expected in the pH and HCO_3 levels?

Answer: pH _____

HCO₃ _____

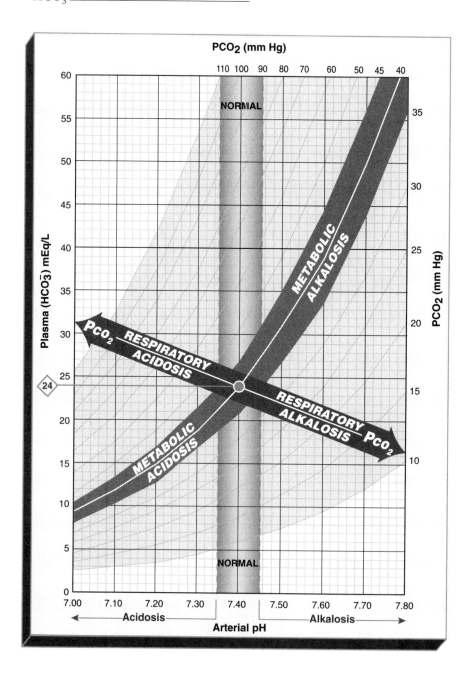

2. List common causes of **acute ventilatory failure**.

a. _____

b. _____

c. _____

d. _____

e. _____

Renal Compensation

1. Using the P_{CO_2}/HCO_3/pH nomogram provided below, if a patient has a Pa_{CO_2} of 70 mm Hg, at a time when the pH is 7.30 and the HCO_3 is 33, the patient's acid-base status would be called
   a. acute ventilatory failure
   b. acute ventilatory failure (with partial renal compensation)
   c. chronic ventilatory failure (with complete renal compensation)
   d. acute alveolar hyperventilation
   e. acute alveolar hyperventilation (with partial renal compensation)
   f. chronic alveolar hyperventilation (with complete renal compensation)

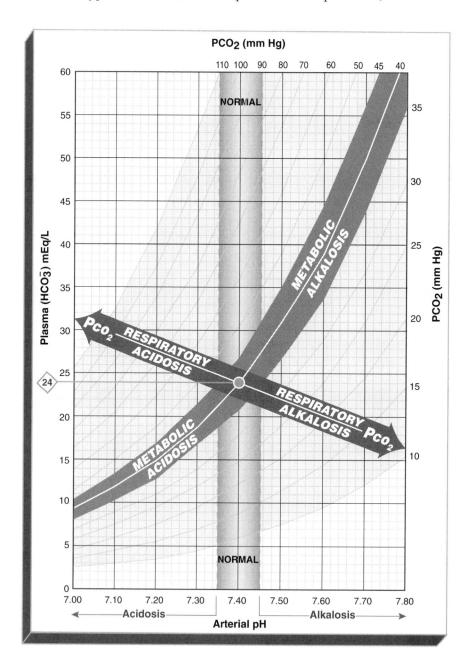

2. In regard to the case shown, the HCO_3 would need to increase, or decrease, to about what level in order to correct the pH (i.e., 7.35 or greater)?

Answer: _____

Acute Alveolar Hyperventilation (Respiratory Alkalosis)

1. Using the P_{CO_2}/HCO_3/pH nomogram provided below, if a patient's ventilatory rate suddenly increased and caused the patient's Pa_{CO_2} to increase to 20 mm Hg, what approximate changes would be expected in the pH and HCO_3 levels?

Answer: pH _____

   HCO_3 _____

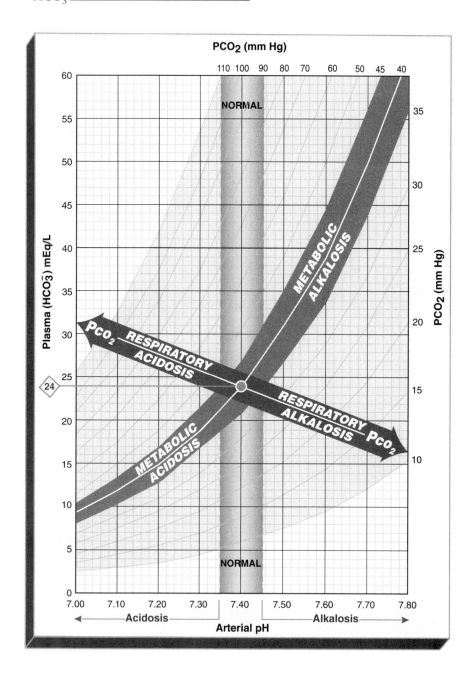

2. List common causes of acute alveolar hyperventilation.

    a. _____

    b. _____

    c. _____

    d. _____

Renal Compensation

1. Using the P_{CO_2}/HCO_3/pH nomogram provided below, if a patient has a Pa_{CO_2} of 25 mm Hg, at a time when the pH is 7.50 and the HCO_3 is 19, the patient's acid-base status would be called
   a. acute ventilatory failure
   b. acute ventilatory failure (with partial renal compensation)
   c. chronic ventilatory failure (with complete renal compensation)
   d. acute alveolar hyperventilation
   e. acute alveolar hyperventilation (with partial renal compensation)
   f. chronic alveolar hyperventilation (with complete renal compensation)

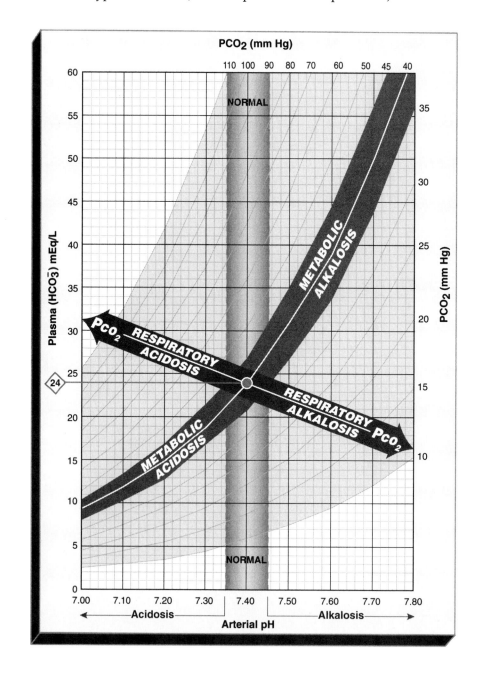

2. In regard to the case shown, the HCO_3 would need to increase, or decrease, to about what level in order to correct the pH (i.e., 7.45 or less)?

Answer: _____

Metabolic Acid-Base Imbalances

Metabolic Acidosis

1. Using the P_{CO_2}/HCO_3/pH nomogram provided below, if a patient's Pa_{CO_2} is 40 mm Hg at a time when the pH is 7.14, what is the expected HCO_3 level?

Answer: HCO_3 _____

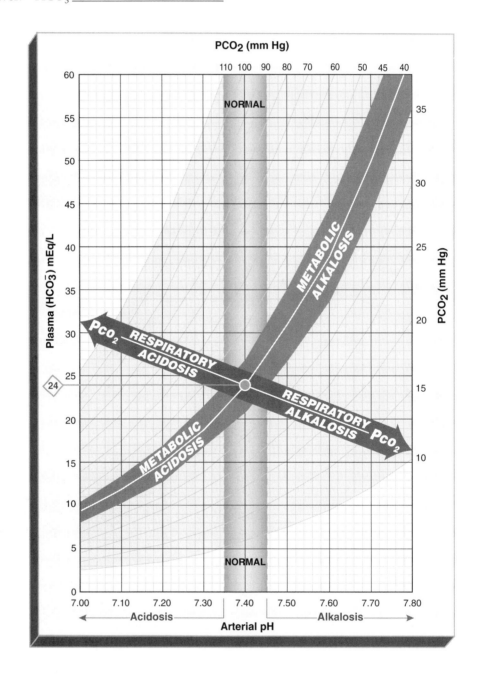

2. List common causes of **metabolic acidosis**.

a. _____

b. _____

c. _____

d. _____

e. _____

Anion Gap

1. Identify the normal plasma concentrations of the following cations and anions:

a. Na^+: _____

b. Cl^-: _____

c. HCO_3^-: _____

2. What is a patient's **anion gap** with the following clinical data:
a. Na^+: 132 mEq/L
b. Cl^-: 97 mEq/L
c. HCO_3^-: 22 mEq/L

Answer: _____

3. An anion gap greater than _____ represents acidosis.

4. An elevated anion gap is most commonly caused by the accumulation of _____ .

5. Metabolic acidosis caused by a decreased HCO_3^- is often called _____ .

Metabolic Acidosis with Respiratory Compensation

1. Using the $P_{CO_2}/HCO_3/pH$ nomogram provided below, if a patient has a Pa_{CO_2} of 20 mm Hg, at a time when the pH is 7.28 and the HCO_3 is 9, the patient's acid-base status would be called
   a. metabolic acidosis
   b. metabolic acidosis (with partial respiratory compensation)
   c. metabolic acidosis (with complete respiratory compensation)
   d. both metabolic and respiratory acidosis
   e. metabolic alkalosis
   f. metabolic alkalosis (with partial respiratory compensation)
   g. metabolic alkalosis (with complete respiratory compensation)
   h. both metabolic and respiratory acidosis

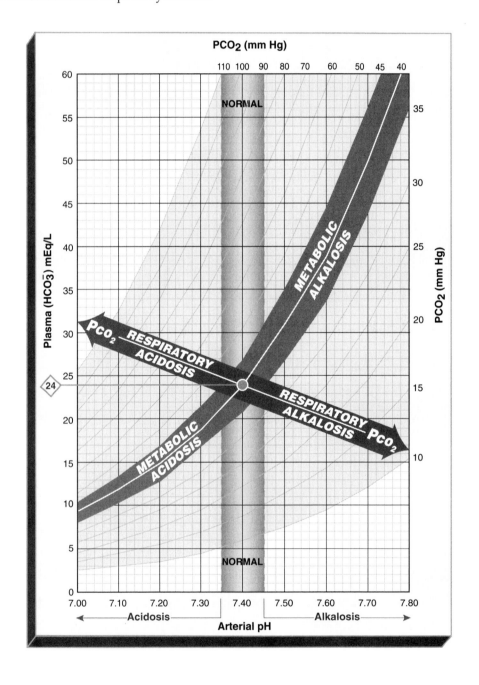

2. In regard to the case shown, the Pa_{CO_2} would need to increase, or decrease, to about what level in order to correct the pH (i.e., 7.35 or greater)?

Answer: _____

3. Using the P_{CO_2}/HCO_3/pH nomogram provided below, if a patient has a Pa_{CO_2} of 90 mm Hg, at a time when the pH is 7.04 and the HCO_3 is 24, the patient's acid-base status would be called

    a. metabolic acidosis

    b. metabolic acidosis (with partial respiratory compensation)

    c. metabolic acidosis (with complete respiratory compensation)

    d. both metabolic and respiratory acidosis

    e. metabolic alkalosis

    f. metabolic alkalosis (with partial respiratory compensation)

    g. metabolic alkalosis (with complete respiratory compensation)

    h. both metabolic and respiratory alkalosis

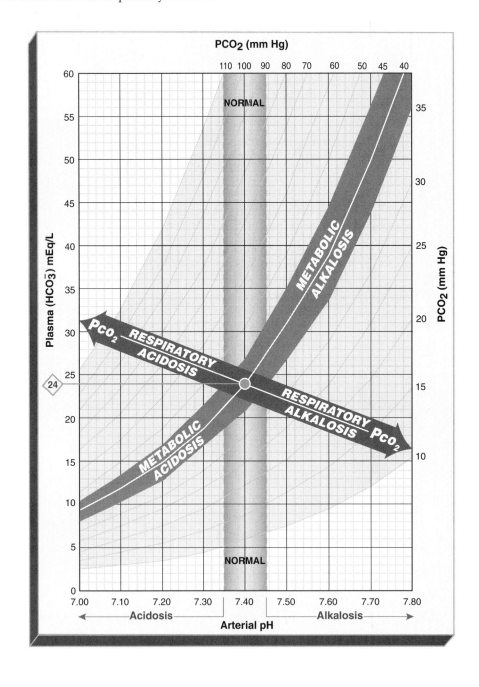

Metabolic Alkalosis

1. Using the P_{CO_2}/HCO_3/pH nomogram provided below, if a patient's Pa_{CO_2} is 40 mm Hg at a time when the pH is 7.60, what is the expected HCO_3 level?

Answer: HCO_3 _____

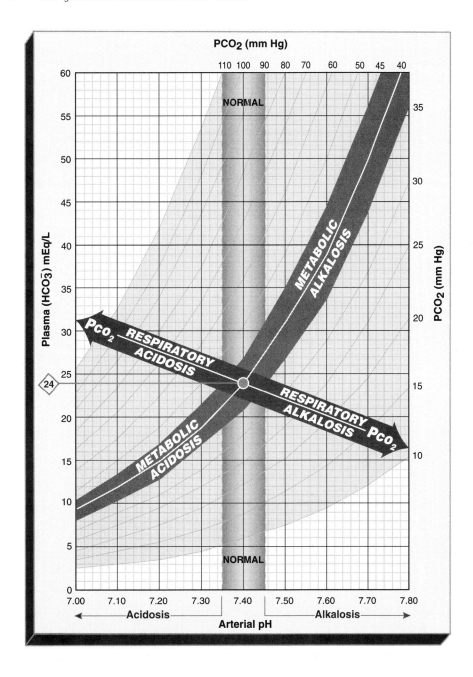

2. List common causes of metabolic alkalosis.

a. _____

b. _____

c. _____

d. _____

e. _____

f. _____

g. _____

Metabolic Alkalosis with Respiratory Compensation

1. Using the P_{CO_2}/HCO_3/pH nomogram provided below, if a patient has a Pa_{CO_2} of 50 mm Hg, at a time when the pH is 7.60 and the HCO_3 is 50, the patient's acid-base status would be called

    a. metabolic acidosis
    b. metabolic acidosis (with partial respiratory compensation)
    c. metabolic acidosis (with complete respiratory compensation)
    d. both metabolic and respiratory acidosis
    e. metabolic alkalosis
    f. metabolic alkalosis (with partial respiratory compensation)
    g. metabolic alkalosis (with complete respiratory compensation)
    h. both metabolic and respiratory alkalosis

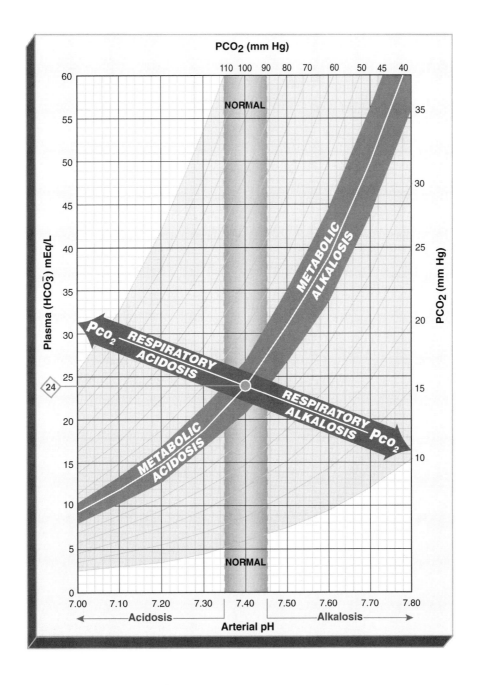

2. In regard to the case shown, the Pa_{CO_2} would need to increase, or decrease, to about what level in order to correct the pH (i.e., 7.45 or less)?

Answer: _____

3. Using the P_{CO_2}/HCO_3/pH nomogram provided below, if a patient had a Pa_{CO_2} of 30 mm Hg, at a time when the pH is 7.60 and the HCO_3 is 29, the patient's acid-base status would be called

   a. metabolic acidosis
   b. metabolic acidosis (with partial respiratory compensation)
   c. metabolic acidosis (with complete respiratory compensation)
   d. both metabolic and respiratory acidosis
   e. metabolic alkalosis
   f. metabolic alkalosis (with partial respiratory compensation)
   g. metabolic alkalosis (with complete respiratory compensation)
   h. both metabolic and respiratory alkalosis

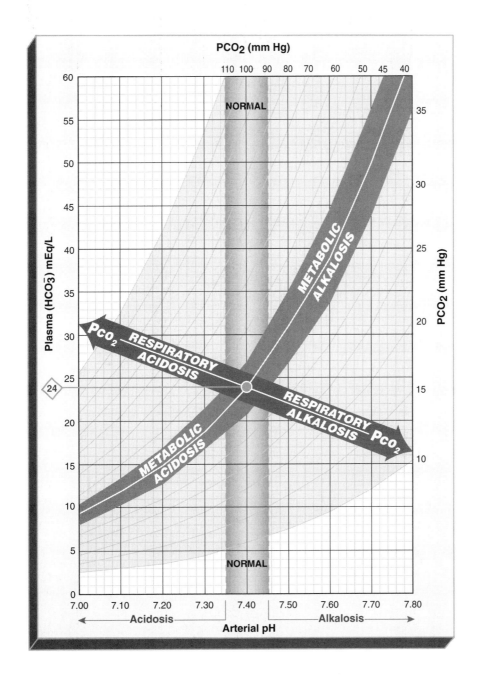

CHAPTER EIGHT

VENTILATION-PERFUSION RELATIONSHIPS

VENTILATION-PERFUSION RATIO

1. The normal alveolar ventilation is about _____ L/min.

2. The normal pulmonary capillary blood flow is about _____ L/min.

3. The average overall **ventilation-perfusion ratio** is _____ to _____ , or _____ .

4. In the normal individual in the upright position, the $\dot{V}/\dot{Q}$ ratio in the upper lung region is

   (_____ higher; _____ lower) than 0.8.

5. In the normal individual in the upright position, the $\dot{V}/\dot{Q}$ ratio in the lower lung region is

   (_____ higher; _____ lower) than 0.8.

6. In the upright lung, the $\dot{V}/\dot{Q}$ ratio progressively (_____ increases; _____ decreases; _____ remains the same) from the top to the bottom.

7. The $P_{A_{O_2}}$ is determined by the balance between

   a. _____

   _____

   b. _____

   _____

8. The $P_{A_{CO_2}}$ is determined by the balance between

   a. _____

   _____

   b. _____

   _____

9. When the $\dot{V}/\dot{Q}$ ratio increases, the $P_{A_{CO_2}}$ decreases because _____

   _____

   _____

   _____

10. When the $\dot{V}/\dot{Q}$ ratio increases, the $P_{A_{O_2}}$ increases because _____

    _____

    _____

    _____

    _____

11. In the upright lung, an increased $\dot{V}/\dot{Q}$ ratio is found in the
    a. upper lung regions
    b. middle lung regions
    c. lower lung regions

12. When the $\dot{V}/\dot{Q}$ ratio decreases, the $P_{A_{O_2}}$ decreases because _____

    _____

    _____

    _____

13. When the $\dot{V}/\dot{Q}$ ratio decreases, the $P_{A_{CO_2}}$ increases because _____

    _____

    _____

    _____

14. In the upright lung, a decreased $\dot{V}/\dot{Q}$ ratio is found in the

   a. upper lung regions
   b. middle lung regions
   c. lower lung regions

15. In the upright lung, the Pc_{O_2} (_____ increases; _____ decreases; _____ remains the same) from the top to the bottom.

16. In the upright lung, the Pc_{CO_2} (_____ increases; _____ decreases; _____ remains the same) from the top to the bottom.

17. In the upright lung, the pH in the end-capillary blood (_____ increases; _____ decreases; _____ remains the same) from the top to the bottom.

18. **Internal respiration** is defined as _____

   _____

   _____

19. Normally, about _____ mL of oxygen are consumed by the tissue cells in 1 minute.

20. Normally, the tissue cells produce about _____ mL of carbon dioxide in 1 minute.

21. **Respiratory quotient** (RQ) is defined as the _____

   _____

   _____

22. The respiratory quotient is expressed as

   RQ =

23. **External respiration** is defined as _____ _____

   _____

   _____

24. **Respiratory exchange ratio** (RR) is defined as the _____

    _____

    _____

25. List some pulmonary disorders that increase the $\dot{V}/\dot{Q}$ ratio:

    a. _____

    _____

    b. _____

    _____

    c. _____

    _____

    d. _____

    _____

    e. _____

    _____

26. List some pulmonary disorders that decrease the $\dot{V}/\dot{Q}$ ratio:

    a. _____

    _____

    b. _____

    _____

    c. _____

    _____

CHAPTER NINE

CONTROL OF VENTILATION

THE RESPIRATORY COMPONENTS OF THE MEDULLA OBLONGATA

1. It is now believed that the DRG and VRG neurons in the medulla oblongata are responsible for coordinating the intrinsic rhythmicity of respiration. DRG and VRG are abbreviations for

   a. DRG: _____

   b. VRG: _____

2. The DRG consists chiefly of

   a. inspiratory neurons
   b. expiratory neurons
   c. inspiratory and expiratory neurons

3. The VRG consists of

   a. inspiratory neurons
   b. expiratory neurons
   c. inspiratory and expiratory neurons

4. Which of the following is activated only during heavy exercise or stress?

   a. DRG
   b. VRG

THE INFLUENCE OF THE PONTINE RESPIRATORY CENTERS ON THE RESPIRATORY COMPONENTS OF THE MEDULLA OBLONGATA

1. Where is the **apneustic center** located? _____

2. If unrestrained, the apneustic center causes

   a. prolonged expiration
   b. prolonged inspiration

3. Which of the following suppresses the function of the apneustic center?

   a. DRG
   b. pneumotaxic center
   c. VRG

MONITORING SYSTEMS THAT INFLUENCE THE RESPIRATORY COMPONENTS OF THE MEDULLA OBLONGATA

1. The respiratory components (DRG and VRG) of the medulla are primarily influenced by an excessive concentration of _____ .

2. Where are the **central chemoreceptors** located? _____

   _____

   _____

3. The **blood-brain barrier** is very permeable to _____ molecules and relatively impermeable

   to _____ and _____ ions.

4. Write the chemical reaction that forms carbonic acid when CO_2 moves into the cerebrospinal fluid:

   $CO_2 +$

5. How do the central chemoreceptors respond to the liberated hydrogen ions [H+] produced in the reaction shown?

_____

_____

_____

_____

6. In essence, the central chemoreceptors regulate ventilation through the (_____ direct; _____ indirect) effects of CO_2 on the _____ .

7. The **peripheral chemoreceptors** are _____

_____

_____

_____

8. Where are the peripheral chemoreceptors located? _____

_____

_____

_____

9. When activated by a low Pa_{O_2}, the carotid bodies send neural impulses to the respiratory components of the medulla by way of the _____ nerve; the aortic bodies send neural impulses to the medulla by way of the _____ nerve.

10. Which of the following play a greater role in causing the ventilatory rate to increase in response to a decreased Pa_{O_2}?

   a. carotid bodies
   b. aortic bodies

11. At about what Pa_{O_2} level are the peripheral chemoreceptors significantly activated?

   Answer: _____

12. Suppression of the peripheral chemoreceptors is seen when the Pa_{O_2} falls below _____

    _____ .

13. Why are the peripheral chemoreceptors totally responsible for the control of ventilation when the Pa_{CO_2} level is chronically high?

    _____

    _____

    _____

    _____

    _____

    _____

    _____

14. In response to a chronically high CO_2 level, the sensitivity of the peripheral chemoreceptors
    a. increases
    b. decreases
    c. remains the same

15. List some clinical conditions in which the P_{O_2} is normal, but the oxygen content is dangerously low:

    a. _____

    b. _____

    c. _____

16. List some other factors that stimulate the peripheral chemoreceptors:

    a. _____

    b. _____

    c. _____

    d. _____

    e. _____

17. In addition to an increase in ventilation, list some other responses that occur when the peripheral chemoreceptors are stimulated:

a. _____

b. _____

c. _____

d. _____

e. _____

REFLEXES THAT INFLUENCE VENTILATION

1. What activates the **Hering-Breuer reflex**? _____

_____

2. When activated, the Hering-Breuer reflex causes _____

_____

3. What activates the **deflation reflex**? _____

_____

4. When activated, the deflation reflex causes _____

_____

5. What activates the **irritant reflex**? _____

_____

_____

6. Where are the irritant receptors located? _____

_____

7. When activated, the irritant reflex causes _____

_____

8. An extensive network of free nerve endings, called **C-fibers**, are located in the _____

_____

_____

9. The C-fibers near the alveolar capillaries are called _____

10. The J-receptors are stimulated by _____

_____

_____

11. When the J-receptors are stimulated, a reflex response triggers a _____

_____

12. **Peripheral proprioceptors** are located in the _____

_____

13. When stimulated, the proprioceptors send neural impulses to the _____

The medulla, in turn, sends out an _____

_____

14. The proprioceptors in the joints and tendons are believed to play a role in initiating and maintaining

an _____

_____

15. The more joints and tendons are involved, the _____ the breathing rate.

16. Strong emotions can activate the centers in the hypothamus; for example, excitement causes the

respiratory rate to (_____ increase, _____ decrease).

17. An increased body temperature causes the respiratory rate to (_____ increase, _____
decrease).

18. In response to an elevated systemic blood pressure, the **aortic and carotid sinus baroreceptors** cause

_____

_____

19. In response to a reduced systemic blood pressure, the aortic and carotid sinus baroreceptors cause

_____

_____

CHAPTER TEN

FETAL DEVELOPMENT AND THE CARDIOPULMONARY SYSTEM

FETAL LUNG DEVELOPMENT

1. List the four periods of lung development during fetal life.

   a. _____

   b. _____

   c. _____

   d. _____

2. The lungs first appear as a small bud arising from the esophagus on the _____ day of embryonic life.

3. By the 16th week of gestation, there are about _____ generations of bronchial airways.

4. By the _____ week of gestation, the air–blood interface between the alveoli and the pulmonary capillaries and the quantity of pulmonary surfactant are usually sufficient to support life.

PLACENTA

1. Anatomically, the placenta consists of about 15 to 20 segments called _____ .

2. Label and color the following anatomic structures of the placenta:

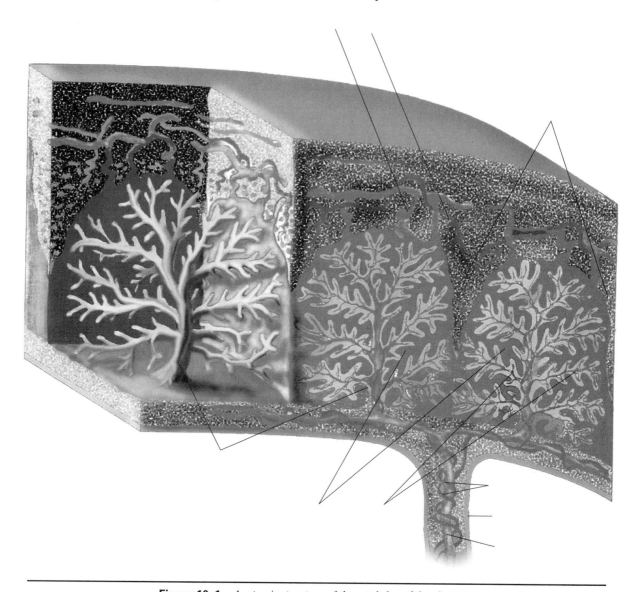

Figure 10–1 *Anatomic structure of the cotyledon of the placenta.*

3. Deoxygenated blood is carried from the fetus to the placenta by way of two _____

_____ .

4. Normally, the P_{O_2} in the umbilical arteries is about _____ mm Hg and the P_{CO_2} is about _____ mm Hg.

5. Explain why the maternal blood P_{CO_2} is frequently lower than expected during the last trimester of pregnancy.

_____

_____

_____

_____

6. Once in the **intervillous space**, oxygen transfers from the maternal to fetal blood because of the

   a. _____

   _____

   b. _____

   _____

   c. _____

   _____

7. As oxygenated fetal blood flows out of the **chorionic villi**, the P_{O_2} is about _____ mm Hg and the P_{CO_2} is about _____ mm Hg.

8. Oxygenated fetal blood flows out of the chorionic villi and returns to the fetus by way of the _____

   _____ .

9. List the three factors thought to be responsible for the wide variance between the maternal and fetal P_{O_2} and P_{CO_2}.

   a. _____

   _____

   b. _____

   _____

   c. _____

   _____

FETAL CIRCULATION

1. As oxygenated blood from the placenta returns to the fetus, about one-half of the blood enters the liver of the fetus and the rest enters the **inferior vena cava** by flowing through the _____ _____ .

2. Once in the **right atrium** of the fetus, most of the blood flows directly into the left atrium through the _____ .

3. The blood in the left atrium of the fetus enters the _____ and is then pumped primarily to the _____ and _____ .

4. Most of the fetal blood that passes into the pulmonary artery from the right ventricle bypasses the lungs by passing through the _____ and flows directly into the _____ .

5. Approximately _____ percent of the fetal circulation passes through the lungs and returns to the left atrium via the _____ .

6. The Pa_{O_2} in the descending aorta is about _____ mm Hg.

7. Directions: In *Column A*, match the order (i.e., from first to last) in which fetal blood passes through the structures in *Column B*.

COLUMN A	COLUMN B
Order	Structure
_____	a. common iliac arteries
_____	b. external and internal iliacs
_____	c. ductus arteriosus
_____	d. umbilical arteries
_____	e. ductus venosus

8. Describe the changes the special structures of the fetal circulation go through after birth:

a. _____

_____

_____

b. _____

_____

_____

c. _____

_____

_____

d. _____

_____

_____

e. _____

_____

_____

f. _____

_____

_____

9. Describe the three primary mechanisms that remove the fluid from the fetal lungs during the first 24 hours of life:

    a. _____

    _____

    _____

    b. _____

    _____

    _____

    c. _____

    _____

    _____

10. About _____ million primitive alveoli are present at birth.

11. The number of alveoli continues to increase until about _____ years of age.

BIRTH

1. List some of the stimuli that cause the infant to take its first breath at birth:

    a. _____

    b. _____

    c. _____

2. During the first breath, it is estimated that the infant's intrapleural pressure decreases to about

    _____ cm H_2O before any air enters the lungs.

3. About _____ mL of air enters the lungs during the first breath.

4. The average lung compliance (C_L) of the newborn is about _____ .

5. The average airway resistance (R_{aw}) of the newborn is about _____ .

6. List the three major mechanisms that account for the decreased pulmonary vascular resistance when an infant inhales for the first time:

   a. _____

   _____

   _____

   b. _____

   _____

   _____

   c. _____

   _____

   _____

7. Describe the mechanism that causes the foramen ovale to close functionally at birth:

   _____

   _____

   _____

   _____

   _____

   _____

   _____

   _____

8. At birth, the newborn's P_{O_2} must increase to more than _____ to _____ mm Hg in order for the ductus arteriosus to close.

9. Describe the meaning of **persistent pulmonary hypertension of the neonate (PPHN)**:

   _____

   _____

   _____

   _____

10. Persistent pulmonary hypertension of the neonate was previously known as _____

_____ .

11. List other substances that are released at birth that are believed to contribute to the constriction of the ductus arteriosus:

    a. _____

    b. _____

    c. _____

CONTROL OF VENTILATION IN THE NEWBORN

1. Although inhibited during fetal life, the _____ and _____

   _____ chemoreceptors play a major role in activating the first breath
   at birth.

2. Stimulation of the newborn's trigeminal nerve causes the infant's respiration and heart rate to

   _____ .

3. Stimulation of the preterm infant's irritant reflex is commonly followed by _____

   _____ .

4. Stimulation of the term infant's irritant reflex causes _____

   _____ .

5. The head paradoxical reflex is _____

   _____ .

CLINICAL PARAMETERS IN THE NORMAL NEWBORN

1. Compare the approximate lung volumes and capacities of the newborn:

TABLE 10–1   Approximate Lung Volumes and Capacities of the Normal Newborn

---

Tidal volume (V_T)   Vital capacity (VC)
Residual volume (RV)   Functional residual capacity (FRC)
Expiratory reserve volume (ERV)   Inspiratory capacity (IC)
Inspiratory reserve volume (IRV)   Total lung capacity (TLC)

---

2. Write the normal vital sign ranges of the newborn:

TABLE 10–2   Vital Sign Ranges of the Normal Newborn

Respiratory rate (RR)
Heart rate (HR)
Blood pressure (BP)

CHAPTER ELEVEN

AGING AND THE CARDIOPULMONARY SYSTEM

THE EFFECTS OF AGING ON THE RESPIRATORY SYSTEM

1. The growth and development of the lungs is essentially complete by about _____ years of age.

2. Most of the pulmonary function indices reach their maximum level between _____ and _____ years of age.

3. With aging, the elastic recoil of the lungs (_____ increases; _____ decreases; _____ remains the same), and the lung compliance (_____ increases; _____ decreases; _____ remains the same).

4. With aging, identify which changes occur (check one) with the following lung volumes and capacities:

    a. RV (_____ increases; _____ decreases; _____ remains the same)

    b. IC (_____ increases; _____ decreases; _____ remains the same)

    c. IC (_____ increases; _____ decreases; _____ remains the same)

    d. TLC (_____ increases; _____ decreases; _____ remains the same)

    e. RV/TLC (_____ increases; _____ decreases; _____ remains the same)

    f. FRC (_____ increases; _____ decreases; _____ remains the same)

    g. ERV (_____ increases; _____ decreases; _____ remains the same)

5. With aging, identify which changes occur with the following dynamic maneuvers of ventilation:

   a. FVC (_____ increases; _____ decreases; _____ remains the same)

   b. PEFR (_____ increases; _____ decreases; _____ remains the same)

   c. $FEF_{25\%-75\%}$ (_____ increases; _____ decreases; _____ remains the same)

   d. FEV_1 (_____ increases; _____ decreases; _____ remains the same)

   e. FEV_1/FVC ratio (_____ increases; _____ decreases; _____ remains the same)

   f. FRC (_____ increases; _____ decreases; _____ remains the same)

   g. MVV (_____ increases; _____ decreases; _____ remains the same)

6. With aging, identify which changes occur with the following components of the respiratory system:

   a. Pulmonary diffusing capacity (_____ increases; _____ decreases; _____ remains the same)

   b. Alveolar deadspace ventilation (_____ increases; _____ decreases; _____ remains the same)

   c. $P(A - a)_{O_2}$ (_____ increases; _____ decreases; _____ remains the same)

   d. Pa_{O_2} (_____ increases; _____ decreases; _____ remains the same)

   e. Pa_{CO_2} (_____ increases; _____ decreases; _____ remains the same)

   f. HCO_3^- (_____ increases; _____ decreases; _____ remains the same)

   g. pH (_____ increases; _____ decreases; _____ remains the same)

   h. $C(a - \bar{v})_{O_2}$ (_____ increases; _____ decreases; _____ remains the same)

   i. Hemoglobin concentration (_____ increases; _____ decreases; _____ remains the same)

ARTERIAL BLOOD GASES

1. With aging, the ventilatory response to both hypoxia and hypercapnia

   a. increases
   b. decreases
   c. remains the same

2. With aging, the

    a. mucocilary transport system (_____ increases; _____ decreases; _____ remains the same)

    b. cough reflex (_____ increases; _____ decreases; _____ remains the same)

3. With aging, the maximal oxygen uptake ($\dot{V}_{O_2}$ max)

    a. increases
    b. decreases
    c. remains the same

THE EFFECTS OF AGING ON THE CARDIOVASCULAR SYSTEM

1. With aging, the elasticity of the heart

    a. increases
    b. decreases
    c. remains the same

2. With aging, the work of the heart

    a. increases
    b. decreases
    c. remains the same

3. With aging, the heart rate reacts as follows in response to stress:

    a. is more likely to increase dramatically
    b. is less likely to increase dramatically
    c. remains the same

4. What is the maximum heart rate for a 70-year-old?

    Answer: _____

5. With aging, identify which changes develop (check one) with the following components of the cardiovascular system:

   a. Stroke volume (_____ increases; _____ decreases; _____ remains the same)

   b. Cardiac output (_____ increases; _____ decreases; _____ remains the same)

   c. Resting pulse pressure (_____ increases; _____ decreases; _____ remains the same)

   d. Systolic blood pressure (_____ increases; _____ decreases; _____ remains the same)

   e. Peripheral vascular resistance (_____ increases; _____ decreases; _____ remains the same)

   f. Aerobic capacity (_____ increases; _____ decreases; _____ remains the same)

Section II
ADVANCED CARDIOPULMONARY CONCEPTS AND RELATED AREAS—THE ESSENTIALS

CHAPTER TWELVE

ELECTROPHYSIOLOGY OF THE HEART

ELECTROPHYSIOLOGY OF THE HEART

1. The way in which the heart contracts is by generating and propagating _____ .

2. When the heart is relaxed (i.e., not generating an action potential), the cardiac muscle fibers are in what is called their _____ or _____ .

3. When the heart is relaxed, there is an electrical charge difference across the fibers of the heart cells. This electrical difference between the electrolytes inside the cell membranes and the electrolytes outside of the cell membranes is called the _____ .

4. The primary electrolytes responsible for the electrical difference across the RMP are _____ .

5. When the heart is relaxed, the concentration of K^+ is (_____ lowest, _____ greatest) inside the cardiac cell.

6. When the cardiac cell is relaxed, the inside of the cell is negatively charged with the _____ and the outside of the cell is positively charged with the _____ .

7. The RMP of the myocardial cells is about _____ .

8. A cornerstone to the understanding of the electrophysiology of the heart are the five electrophysiologic phases of the _____ .

THE FIVE PHASES OF THE ACTION POTENTIAL

1. During phase 0, an electrical impulse is initiated by the sinoatrial (SA) node. This action changes the RMP and allows a rapid inward flow of _____ into the cell through specific _____ . This process causes the inside of the cell to become _____ .

2. The voltage inside the cell at the end of **depolarization** is about _____ . This electrophysiologic event produces a rapid (_____ down-stroke; _____ up-stroke) in the action potential.

3. Immediately after phase 0, phase 1 starts. During this period the channels for _____ open and permit _____ to flow (____ in; ____ out) of the cell.

4. Phase 1 is illustrated as a short (____ downward; ____ upward) stroke in the action potential curve just before the plateau.

5. During phase 2, there is a slow (____ inward; ____ outward) flow of _____ , which in turn slows the (____ inward; ____ outward) flow of _____ significantly.

6. During the **plateau phase**, the contraction of the myocardial cells is (____ prolonged; ____ shortened).

7. During phase 3, the (_____ inward; _____ outward) flow of _____ stops, and the (_____ inward; _____ outward) flow of ____ is again accelerated, and the rate of repolarization accelerates.

8. During phase 4, the excess ____ inside the cell and the loss of ____ are returned to normal by the ____ and ____ ion pumps.

PROPERTIES OF THE CARDIAC MUSCLE

1. The heart is composed of two types of cardiac cells: the _____ and the specialized "pacemaker cells" called the _____ .

2. The myocardial _____ make up the bulk of the musculature of the myocardium and are responsible for the pumping activity of the heart.

3. The majority of the autorhythmic cells are located in the _____ .

4. **Automaticity** is the unique ability of the cells in the sinoatrial (SA) node (pacemaker cells) to generate an action potential without being stimulated. This is because the cell membranes of the pacemaker cells permit Na^+ to leak (____ into; ____ out of) the cell during phase ____ .

5. **Excitability** (irritability) is the ability of a cell to reach its threshold potential and respond to a stimulus or irritation. The lower the stimulus needed to activate a cell, the (____ less; ____ more) excitable the cell; the greater the stimulus needed, the (____ less; ____ more) excitable the cell.

6. **Conductivity** is the unique ability of the heart cells to _____ electrical current from _____ throughout the entire conductive system.

7. **Contractility** is the ability of cardiac muscle fibers to _____ in response to an electrical stimulus.

Refractory Periods

1. The **absolute refractory period** is the time in which the cells _____

_____ .

2. Phases _____ represent the absolute refractory period.

3. The **relative refractory period** is the time in which repolarization is almost complete and a _____ stimulus may cause depolarization.

4. The second half of phase ____ represents the relative refractory period of the action potential.

5. The **nonrefractory period** occurs when all the cells are in their _____

_____ .

6. Phase ____ represents the nonrefractory period.

The Conductive System

1. Using the following illustration, label the components of the conductive system of the heart:

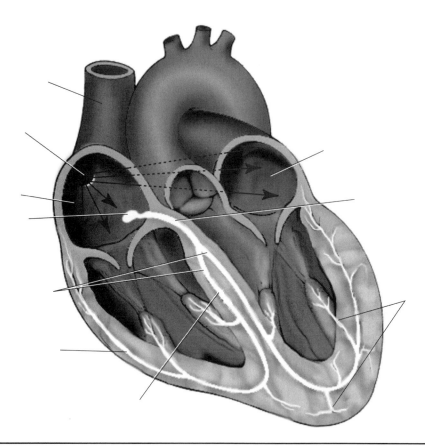

Figure 12–1 *Conductive system of the heart.*

Autonomic Nervous System

1. **Sympathetic** neural fibers innervate the atria and ventricles of the heart. When stimulated, the

   sympathetic fibers cause an increase in the _____

   _____ .

2. Stimulation of the **parasympathetic** system causes a decrease in the _____

   _____ .

CHAPTER THIRTEEN

THE STANDARD 12-ECG SYSTEM

THE STANDARD 12-ECG SYSTEM

1. The standard 12-ECG system consists of _____ limb electrodes and _____ chest electrodes.

2. In Table 13-1, list the 6 standard limb leads (bipolar and unipolar) and the 6 precordial (chest) leads.

TABLE 13-1   ECG Lead Systems

STANDARD LIMB LEADS		PRECORDIAL (CHEST) LEADS
Bipolar Leads	Unipolar Leads	Unipolar Leads

3. Each lead

   a. _____

   b. _____

   c. _____

Standard Limb Leads

1. Leads I, II, and III are _____ , which means they use two electrodes to monitor the heart, one _____ and one _____ .

2. An imaginary line drawn between the positive and negative electrodes for leads I, II, and III represents the _____ of each lead.

3. The triangle formed around the heart by the three axes is called _____ _____ .

4. Electrical impulses that travel more toward the positive electrode (relative to the axis of the lead) are recorded as _____ .

5. When an electrical current travels perpendicular to the lead axis, an _____ or _____ line is recorded.

6. Electrical impulses that move away from the positive electrode (or more toward the negative electrode) are recorded as _____ deflections in that lead.

7. In the normal heart, the largest electrical impulse travels from the _____ of the heart to the _____ , in a _____ to _____ direction.

8. **Unipolar leads** monitor the electrical activity of the heart between the _____ electrode and the _____ electrical reference point at the _____ of the heart. In essence, the _____ of the heart functions as a _____ electrode. Thus, the axis for these leads is drawn from the _____ and the _____ of the heart.

9. When the negative electrodes are eliminated in the aVR, aVL, and aVF, the amplitude of the ECG recordings are augmented by _____ . This is the reason for the letter *a*, which stands for _____ . The *V* represents _____ . The letters *R*, *L*, and *F* represent where the _____ .

10. Collectively, the limb leads monitor the electrical activity of the heart in the _____ , which is the electrical activity that flows over the anterior surface of the heart; from the _____ , in a _____ to _____ direction.

11. Leads I and aVL are called _____ , because they monitor the left lateral side of the heart. Leads II, III, and aVF view the lower surfaces of the heart and

called the _____ .

Precordial (Chest) Leads

1. The precordial leads monitor the heart from the _____ , which means they record electrical activity that transverses through the heart. Leads V1 and V2 monitor the

_____ . V3 and V4 monitor the _____ ,

and V5 and V6 view the _____ .

2. Leads V1, V2, V3, and V4 are also called the _____ . Leads V5 and V6 are also called

the _____ .

Modified Chest Lead

1. The modified chest lead (MCL_1) is a _____ bipolar chest lead similar to the precordial lead.

The positive electrode is on the chest and the negative electrode is on the _____

_____ .

NORMAL ECG CONFIGURATIONS AND THEIR EXPECTED MEASUREMENTS (LEAD II)

The ECG Paper

1. All ECG systems use the same standard paper and run at the same speed. Each **small square** has

a duration of _____ second. Each **large square**, delineated by the darker lines, has

_____ small squares, and a duration of _____ second.

2. The paper on all ECG monitors run at a speed of _____ large squares per second, or

_____ large squares per minute.

3. The vertical portion of each small square also represents an _____ (or voltage) of

_____ **millivolt** (mV), and _____ **millimeter** in distance.

4. Prior to each test, the ECG monitor is standardized so that 1 mV is equal to _____ mm.

5. Most ECG paper has small vertical line marks in the margins every _____ large squares, or every _____ seconds.

6. A single waveform begins and ends at the _____ . When the waveform continues past the baseline, _____ .

7. Two or more waveforms together are a _____ .

8. A flat, straight, or isoelectric line is called a _____ .

9. A waveform, or complex, connected to a segment is called an _____ .

10. All ECG tracings above the baseline are described as _____ deflections. Waveforms below the baseline are _____ deflections.

The P Wave

1. The normal cycle of electrical activity in the heart begins with atrial depolarization and is recorded as the _____ .

2. The shape of the P wave is usually _____ and _____ .

3. The P wave is followed by a short pause while the electrical current passes through the _____ .

4. This is seen on the ECG tracing as a _____ , or _____ , line after the P wave.

5. The normal duration of the P wave is _____ to _____ second, or _____ small horizontal squares.

6. The normal amplitude of the P wave is _____ to _____ mV, or _____ small vertical squares.

7. An increased duration or amplitude of the P wave indicates _____ .

8. Repolarization of the atria is usually not recorded on an ECG tracing. This is because atrial repolarization normally occurs when the _____ .

The PR Interval

1. The PR interval starts at the beginning of the _____ and ends at the beginning of the _____ .

2. The normal duration of the PR interval is _____ to _____ second, or

   _____ to _____ small horizontal squares.

3. The PR interval represents the total atrial (supraventricular) electrical activity prior to the activation

   of the _____ , _____ , and _____

   _____ .

The QRS Complex

1. The QRS complex represents _____ .

2. The QRS complex consists of three separate waves forms: the _____ , _____ , and

   _____ .

3. The first negative defection (below the baseline) after the P wave is the _____ .

4. The next tall positive deflection (above the baseline) is the _____ .

5. The _____ wave is the small negative deflection (below the baseline) that follows the **R wave**.

6. Under normal conditions, the duration of the QRS complex is less than _____ second, or

   _____ small squares.

7. Abnormal ventricular-induced QRS complex waves are (_____ longer; _____ shorter) than

   _____ second.

8. Other characteristics of an abnormal QRS complex include _____ ,

   _____ , and _____

   _____ .

The ST Segment

1. The ST segment represents the time between _____ and

   _____ .

2. The ST segment begins at the end of the _____ and ends at the beginning

   of the _____ .

3. Normally, the ST segment measures _____ second or less.

4. A flat, horizontal ST segment above or below the baseline is highly suggestive of _____ .

The T Wave

1. The T wave represents _____

_____ .

2. Normally, the T wave has a positive deflection of about _____ mV.

3. The duration of the T wave normally measures _____ second or less.

4. At the beginning of the T wave, the ventricles are in their effective _____

_____ .

5. At about the peak of the T wave, the ventricles are in their _____ period and, thus, are vulnerable to stimulation.

6. T waves are sensitive indicators for a number of abnormalities, including _____

_____

_____ .

The U Wave

1. The U wave follows the _____ and has the same polarity (deflection) as the

_____ .

2. Because of its low voltage, the U wave usually is _____ .

The QT Interval

1. The QT interval is measured from the beginning of the _____ to the end of the

_____ .

2. The QT interval represents total _____

_____ .

3. The normal QT measures about _____ second.

4. As a general rule, the QT interval should be about _____ of the measured RR interval.

5. The QT interval varies _____ to the heart rate.

CHAPTER FOURTEEN

ECG INTERPRETATION

HOW TO ANALYZE THE WAVEFORMS

Step One: Does the General Appearance of the ECG Tracing Appear Normal or Abnormal?

1. Briefly describe how to assess the general appearance of an ECG for normal or abnormal tracings.

_____

_____

_____

_____

_____

_____

_____

_____

_____

_____

_____

_____

_____

_____

Step Two: Does the Ventricular Activity (QRS Complexes) Appear Normal or Abnormal?

Rate

1. When the ventricular heart rate is **regular**, the rate can be determined by counting the number of

   _____ squares between two consecutive _____ , and then

   dividing _____ by the number of _____ squares.

2. Complete the estimated heart rate per minute for Table 14-1 below:

TABLE 14-1   Calculating Heart Rate by Counting the Number of Large ECG Squares

DISTANCE BETWEEN TWO QRS COMPLEXES (NUMBER OF LARGE SQUARES)	ESTIMATED HEART RATE (PER MIN)
1	
2	
3	
4	
5	
6	

---

3. When the ventricular heart rate is **irregular**, the rate can be calculated by using the

   _____ in the upper margins of the ECG paper.

4. Calculating an irregular heart rate is done by counting the number of QRS complexes in a

   _____ , and then multiplying this number by _____ .

Rhythm

1. The ventricular rhythm is determined by comparing the _____

   RR intervals with the _____ RR intervals.

2. When the time variation between the shortest RR interval and the longest RR interval is greater

than _____ second, the rhythm is irregular.

Shape

1. The normal QRS duration is _____ second or _____ .

2. A QRS complex that is narrow and 0.10 second or less represents a _____

_____ .

3. When the QRS complex is greater than _____ second, and the shape is

_____ , an abnormal electrical source (ectopic focus) is likely to be

present within the ventricle.

Step Three: Does the Atrial Activity Appear Normal or Abnormal?

1. The **rate** of the atrial activity is calculated in the same way as the _____

_____ .

2. Normally, the P wave rate and the QRS rate are _____ .

3. The atrial **rhythm** is calculated in the same way as the _____ ,

except that in this case _____ are used.

4. P wave **shape** abnormalities may include _____

_____

_____

_____

_____

_____ .

Step Four: Does the Atrioventricular Relationship Appear to be Normal?

1. When the AV conduction ratio is greater than 1:1 (e.g., 2:1 or 3:1), not _____

_____

_____ are being conducted to the ventricles.

2. The best method to determine the AV conduction ratio is to ask these two questions:

   a. _____

   b. _____

3. A PR interval greater than _____ second represents an abnormal delay in AV conduction.

Step Five: What Is the ECG Interpretation?

1. Summarize the ECG characteristics of the normal sinus rhythm, as viewed from lead II, given in the left side of the box below:

Normal Sinus Rhythm
P wave
PR interval
QRS complex
QRS rate
QRS rhythm

COMMON CARDIAC DYSRHYTHMIAS

The Sinus Mechanisms

Sinus Bradycardia

1. *Bradycardia* means "_____ heart."

2. In sinus bradycardia, the heart rate is less than _____ beats per minute.

3. Summarize the ECG characteristics of the sinus bradycardia, as viewed from lead II, given in the left side of the box below:

Sinus Bradycardia

P wave

PR interval

QRS complex

QRS rate

QRS rhythm

---

4. Common pathologic causes of sinus bradycardia include _____

_____

_____

_____

_____ .

5. Sinus bradycardia may lead to a _____ cardiac output

and _____ blood pressure.

6. In severe cases, sinus bradycardia may lead to a _____

perfusion and tissue _____ .

Sinus Tachycardia

1. *Tachycardia* means "_____ heart."

2. In sinus tachycardia, the heart rate is between _____ and _____ beats per minute.

3. Summarize the ECG characteristics of the sinus tachycardia, as viewed from lead II, given in the left side of the box below:

Sinus Tachycardia

P wave

PR interval

QRS complex

QRS rate

QRS rhythm

---

4. In the adult, sinus tachycardia is the normal physiologic response to _____

   _____

   _____.

5. Sinus tachycardia is also caused by physiologic stress such as _____

   _____

   _____.

6. Pathologic conditions associated with sinus tachycardia include _____

   _____

   _____.

Sinus Arrhythmia

1. In sinus arrhythmia, the heart rate varies by more than _____ percent.

2. The P-QRS-T pattern is (_____ normal; _____ abnormal).

3. Summarize the ECG characteristics of the sinus arrhythmia, as viewed from lead II, given in the left side of the box below:

Sinus Arrhythmia

P wave

PR interval

QRS complex

QRS rate

QRS rhythm

---

4. A sinus arrhythmia is a normal rhythm in _____

and _____ .

Sinus (SA) Block

1. In a sinus (SA) block, also called a _____ , the SA node initiates

an impulse, but the electrical current through the atria is _____ .

2. When a sinus block occurs, the next P-QRS-T complex appears _____

_____

_____

_____

_____ .

3. Summarize the ECG characteristics of the sinus (SA) block, as viewed from lead II, given in the left side of the box below:

Sinus (SA) Block

P wave

PR interval

QRS complex

QRS rate

QRS rhythm

Sinus Arrest

1. Sinus arrest (SA node arrest) is the _____

   _____

   _____

   _____ .

2. Summarize the ECG characteristics of the sinus arrest, as viewed from lead II, given in the left side of the box below:

Sinus Arrest

P wave

PR interval

QRS complex

QRS rate

QRS rhythm

The Atrial Mechanisms

Premature Atrial Complex

1. A premature atrial complex (PAC) results when _____

   _____

   _____

   _____ .

2. Electrical currents that originate outside the SA node are called _____

   _____ .

3. An ectopic focus in the atria results in a _____ on the ECG tracing.

4. Summarize the ECG characteristics of the premature atrial complex, as viewed from lead II, given in the left side of the box below:

Premature Atrial Complex
P wave
PR interval
QRS complex
QRS rate
QRS rhythm

5. Causes of PACs include _____

   _____

   _____

   _____ .

6. PACs are commonly seen in

   a. _____

   b. _____

Atrial Bigeminy

1. Atrial bigeminy are said to be present is when _____

   _____ .

2. Atrial bigeminy are often one of the first signs of _____

   _____ .

Atrial Tachycardia

1. Atrial tachycardia is present when an atrial ectopic focus depolarizes the atria at a rate of

   _____ to _____ beats per minute.

2. When atrial tachycardia appears suddenly and then disappears moments later, it is referred to as

   _____ .

3. Summarize the ECG characteristics of atrial tachycardia, as viewed from lead II, given in the left side
   of the box below:

Atrial Tachycardia
P' wave
P'R interval
QRS complex
QRS rate
QRS rhythm

4. Atrial tachycardia is associated with conditions that stimulate the sympathetic nervous system, such as _____

_____

_____ .

Atrial Flutter

1. In atrial flutter, the normal P wave is absent and replaced by _____

_____ .

2. Usually, the atrial rate is constant between _____ and _____ beats per minute while the ventricular rate is in the normal range.

3. Summarize the ECG characteristics of atrial flutter, as viewed from lead II, given in the left side of the box below:

Atrial Flutter
ff Waves
P'R interval
QRS complex
QRS rate
QRS rhythm

4. Atrial flutter is frequently seen in patients over _____ years of age with _____

_____

_____

_____ .

Atrial Fibrillation

1. Atrial fibrillation is a chaotic, _____

   _____

   _____ .

2. Atrial fibrillation is usually easy to identify and is often referred to as _____

   _____ .

3. The atrial rate cannot be measured, as it often reaches rates between _____ and

   _____ beats per minute.

4. The atrial P′ waves are called _____ or _____ .

5. Summarize the ECG characteristics of atrial fibrillation given in the left side of the box below:

Atrial Fibrillation
ff waves
PR interval
QRS complex
QRS rate
QRS rhythm

6. Atrial fibrillation is associated with _____

   _____

   _____

   _____ .

7. Paroxysmal atrial fibrillation may also occur as a result of _____

_____

_____ .

The Ventricular Mechanisms

Premature Ventricular Complex (PVC)

1. A premature ventricular complex (PVC) is the result of _____

_____

_____ .

2. Summarize the ECG characteristics of the premature ventricular complex given in the left side of the box below:

Premature Ventricular Complex

P wave

PR interval

QRS complex

QRS rate

QRS rhythm

---

3. PVCs may occur in various forms, including _____ ,

_____ , _____ ,

_____ , and _____ .

4. *Uniform PVCs* (also called unifocal) orginate _____ . All the PVCs on

an ECG tracing are similar in _____ .

5. *Multiform PVCs* (also called multifocal) originate from _____

_____ . When this occurs, the PVCs take on different

_____ .

6. *Paired PVCs* (also called couplets) are _____ .

7. Ventricular *bigeminy* is a PVC _____

_____

_____ .

8. *Trigeminy* is _____

_____ .

9. Common causes of PVCs include _____

_____

_____

_____ .

10. PVCs may also develop as a result of certain medications such as _____

_____

_____

_____ .

Ventricular Tachycardia

1. Three or more PVCs occurring in a row represent _____

_____ .

2. The rate is regular, or slightly irregular, between _____ and _____ beats per minute.

3. When ventricular tachycardia appears suddenly and then disappears moments later, it is referred

   to as _____ or _____ ventricular tachycardia.

4. When the ECG tracing shows only ventricular tachycardia, it is called _____

   _____ or _____ .

5. The patient's blood pressure is often (_____ increased; _____ decreased) during ventricular tachycardia.

6. Summarize the ECG characteristics of ventricular tachycardia given in the left side of the box below:

Ventricular Tachycardia

P wave

PR interval

QRS complex

QRS rate

QRS rhythm

Ventricular Flutter

1. In ventricular flutter, the EEG shows poorly defined _____ .

2. The rate is _____ to _____ beats per minute.

3. Summarize the ECG characteristics of ventricular flutter given in the left side of the box below:

Ventricular Flutter

P wave

PR interval

QRS complex

QRS rate

QRS rhythm

Ventricular Fibrillation

1. Ventricular fibrillation is characterized by _____

    _____

    _____ .

2. Ventricular fibrillation is a _____ rhythm.

3. Summarize the ECG characteristics of ventricular fibrillation given in the left side of the box below:

Ventricular Fibrillation

P wave

PR interval

QRS complex

QRS rate

QRS rhythm

Asystole (Cardiac Standstill)

1. Asystole is the _____

   _____

   _____ .

2. The ECG tracing appears as _____ and indicates

   _____

   _____

   _____ .

AV Conduction Defects

Sinus Rhythm with First-Degree AV Block

1. When the atrial impulse is delayed as it moves through the AV node, the PR interval (_____

   _____ increases; _____ decreases).

2. When the PR interval is consistently greater than 0.20 second, a _____

   _____ is said to exist.

3. Summarize the ECG characteristics of first-degree AV block, as viewed from lead II, given in the left
   side of the box below:

First-degree AV Block

P wave

PR interval

QRS complex

QRS rate

QRS rhythm

---

4. Causes of first-degree AV blocks include _____

_____

_____ .

Sinus Rhythm with Second-Degree AV Block: The Wenckebach Phenomenon

1. The **Wenckebach phenomenon** is a _____

_____

_____

_____ .

2. Summarize the ECG characteristics of the Wenckebach phenomenon in the space below:

_____

_____

_____

_____

_____

_____

_____

_____

Complete AV Block

1. When the pathology of the AV junction is severe, all the sinus impulses may be _____

_____ .

2. When a **complete AV block** is present, the _____ takes

control of the ventricular rhythm at a rate of _____ to

_____ beats per minute. This mechanism is referred as the

_____ .

3. When the complete AV block is caused by pathology below the bundle of His, the ventricular

   rhythm is controlled by what is called a _____

   _____

   _____ .

4. The rate of the ventricular escape mechanism is between _____ and

   _____ beats per minute.

5. Summarize the ECG characteristics of complete AV block, as viewed from lead II, given in the left
   side of the box below:

Complete AV Block

P wave

PR interval

QRS complex

QRS rate

QRS rhythm

CHAPTER FIFTEEN

HEMODYNAMIC MEASUREMENTS

HEMODYNAMIC MEASUREMENTS DIRECTLY OBTAINED BY MEANS OF THE PULMONARY ARTERY CATHETER

1. **Hemodynamics** is defined as _____

_____

_____

2. Write the abbreviation and normal range for the following hemodynamic values directly obtained by means of the pulmonary artery catheter:

TABLE 15–1 **Hemodynamic Values Directly Obtained by Means of the Pulmonary Artery Catheter**

HEMODYNAMIC VALUE	ABBREVIATION	NORMAL RANGE
Central venous pressure		
Right atrial pressure		
Mean pulmonary artery pressure		
Pulmonary capillary wedge pressure (also called pulmonary artery wedge; pulmonary artery occlusion)		
Cardiac output		

HEMODYNAMIC VALUES COMPUTED FROM DIRECT MEASUREMENTS

1. Write the abbreviation and normal range for the following computed hemodynamic values:

TABLE 15–2   Computed Hemodynamic Values

HEMODYNAMIC VARIABLE	ABBREVIATION	NORMAL RANGE
Stroke volume		
Stroke volume index		
Cardiac index		
Right ventricular stroke work index		
Left ventricular stroke work index		
Pulmonary vascular resistance		
Systemic vascular resistance		

2. **Stroke volume** (SV) is defined as _____

_____

_____

3. List the major determinants of stroke volume:

   a. _____

   b. _____

   c. _____

4. Complete the following equation:

   SV =

5. If a patient has a cardiac output of 5.5 L/min and a heart rate of 87 beats/min, what is the stroke volume?

Answer: _____

6. Fill in factors that increase and decrease the following hemodynamic variables:

TABLE 15–3   Factors Increasing and Decreasing Stroke Volume (SV), Stroke Volume Index (SVI), Cardiac Output (CO), Cardiac Index (CI), Right Ventricular Stroke Work Index (RVSWI), and Left Ventricular Stroke Work Index (LVSWI)

INCREASES	DECREASES
Positive Inotropic Drugs (Increased Contractility)	Negative Inotropic Drugs (Decreased Contractility)
Abnormal Conditions	Abnormal Conditions
	Hyperinflation of Lungs

7. The **stroke volume index** (SVI) is derived by _____
_____
_____

8. If a patient has a stroke volume of 55 mL and a body surface area of 2.5 m², what is the SVI?

Answer: _____

9. Clinically, what does the SVI reflect?

   a. _____

   b. _____

   c. _____

10. The **cardiac index** (CI) is calculated by _____

    _____

    _____

11. If a patient has a cardiac output of 7 L/min and a body surface area of 2.5 m^2, what is the CI?

    Answer: _____

12. What does the **right ventricular stroke work index** (RVSWI) measure?

    _____

    _____

    _____

13. Clinically, what does the RVSWI reflect?

    _____

    _____

14. Complete the following equation:

    RVSWI =

15. If a patient has a SVI of 40 mL/beat/m^2, a PA of 25 mm Hg, and a CVP of 10 mm Hg, what is the RVSWI?

    Answer: _____

16. What does the **left ventricular stroke work index** (LVSWI) measure?

    _____

    _____

    _____

17. Clinically, what does the LVSWI reflect?

    _____

    _____

18. Complete the following equation:

    LVSWI =

19. If a patient has an SVI of 45 mL/beat/m^2, an MAP of 125 mm Hg, and a PCWP of 10 mm Hg, what is the LVSWI?

    Answer: _____

20. The pulmonary vascular system is a (_____ high-; _____ low-) resistance system.

21. The systemic vascular system is a (_____ high-; _____ low-) resistance system.

22. Clinically, what does **pulmonary vascular resistance** (PVR) indicate?

    Answer: _____

23. Complete the following equation:

    PVR =

24. If a patient has a $\overline{PA}$ of 20, a PCWP of 10 mm Hg, and a CO of 7 L/min, what is the PVR?

    Answer: _____

25. Clinically, what does **systemic vascular resistance** (SVR) indicate?

    Answer: _____

26. Complete the following equation:

    SVR =

27. If a patient has an MAP of 105 mm Hg, a CVP of 10 mm Hg, and a CO of 6 L/min, what is the SVR?

    Answer: _____

28. Fill in under each category below the factors that increase pulmonary vascular resistance:

TABLE 15–4   Factors That Increase Pulmonary Vascular Resistance (PVR)

Chemical Stimuli   Pathologic Factors

Pharmacologic Agents

Hyperinflation of Lungs

                                                  Humoral Substances

---

29. Fill in under the categories below factors that decrease pulmonary vascular resistance (PVR):

TABLE 15–5   **Factors That Decrease Pulmonary Vascular Resistance (PVR)**

Pharmacologic Agents	Humoral Substances

30. Fill in under the categories below factors that increase and decrease systemic vascular resistance (SVR):

TABLE 15–6   **Factors That Increase and Decrease Systemic Vascular Resistance (SVR)**

INCREASES SVR	DECREASES SVR
Vasoconstricting Agents	Vasodilating Agents
Abnormal Conditions	Abnormal Conditions

CHAPTER SIXTEEN

RENAL FAILURE AND ITS EFFECTS ON THE CARDIOPULMONARY SYSTEM

THE KIDNEYS

1. Label and color the following structures that form the **kidney**:

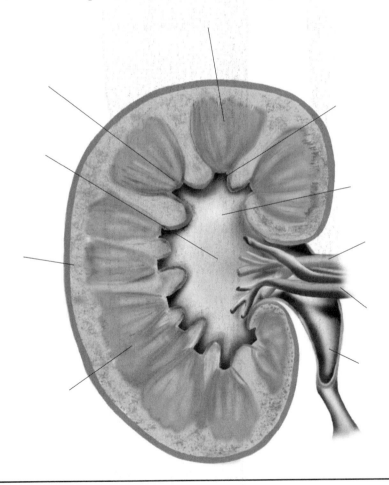

Figure 16–1 *Cross-section of the kidney.*

2. Label and color the following structures of the **nephron**:

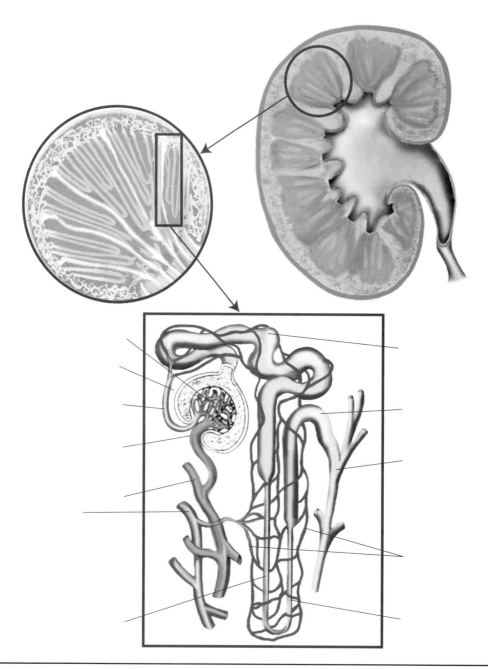

Figure 16–2 *The nephron.*

3. Label and color the following **blood vessels** of the kidney:

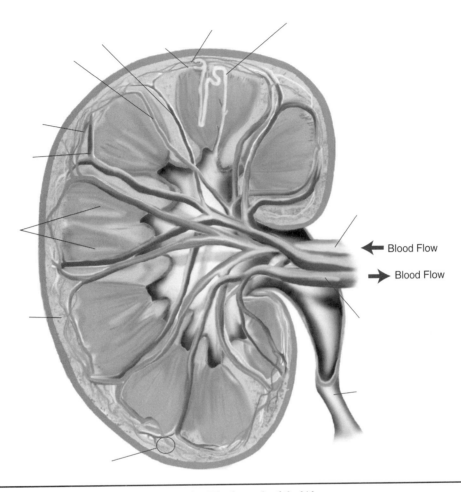

Blood Flow

Blood Flow

Figure 16–3   *Blood vessels of the kidney.*

URINE FORMATION

1. Compare the forces of glomerular filtration:

TABLE 16–1   Forces of Glomerular Filtration

FACTORS	FORCE
Enhances Filtration	
Glomerular capillary blood pressure	
Opposes Filtration	
Fluid pressure in Bowman's capsule	
Osmotic force (caused by the protein concentration difference)	_____
Net Filtration Pressure	

2. List the three major structures responsible for tubular reabsorption:

   a. _____

   b. _____

   c. _____

3. The bulk of tubular reabsorption occurs in the _____

   _____ .

4. Tubular secretion is the mechanism by which _____

   _____

   _____

   _____

   _____

5. The most important substances transported into the tubules by means of secretion are

   _____ and _____ ions.

URINE CONCENTRATION AND VOLUME

1. The kidneys control the concentration and volume of urine by virtue of the following two mechanisms:

   a. _____

   b. _____

   _____

2. The **juxtamedullary nephrons** are located deep into the _____

   _____ .

3. The normal osmolality of the glomerular filtrate is approximately _____ mOsm/L.

4. The osmolality of the interstitial fluid ranges from about _____ mOsm/L in the cortex to about

   _____ mOsm/L as the juxtamedullary nephron descends into the renal medulla.

5. ADH is produced in the _____ and is released by the

   _____ .

6. When the atrial blood volume and pressure increase, the production of ADH

   a. increases
   b. decreases
   c. remains the same

7. When the production of ADH decreases, the volume of urine (_____ increases; _____ decreases).

8. When the atrial blood volume and pressure decrease, the production of ADH

   a. increases
   b. decreases
   c. remains the same

9. When the production of ADH increases, the volume of urine (_____ increases; _____ decreases).

10. The urine produced by the healthy kidney has a specific gravity of about _____ to

    _____ .

REGULATION OF ELECTROLYTE CONCENTRATION

1. List some of the more important ions regulated by the kidneys:

    a. _____

    b. _____

    c. _____

    _____

    _____

ROLE OF THE KIDNEYS IN ACID-BASE BALANCE

1. When the extracellular fluid becomes too acidic, the kidneys excrete _____ ions into the urine.

2. When the extracellular fluid becomes too alkaline, the kidneys excrete (primarily) _____

    _____ into the urine.

BLOOD VOLUME

1. The two major mechanisms responsible for maintaining an individual's blood volume at a consistent level are

    a. _____

    b. _____

RENAL FAILURE

1. List some congenital renal disorders:

   a. _____

   b. _____

   c. _____

2. Urinary tract infections are seen more often in (_____ men; _____ women).

3. List some factors that predispose an individual to urinary flow obstruction:

   a. _____

   b. _____

   c. _____

   d. _____

   e. _____

4. List some causes of kidney inflammation:

   a. _____

   b. _____

   c. _____

5. Name the form of cancer that accounts for about 70 percent of all cancers of early childhood.

   Answer: _____

6. List some common prerenal causes of renal failure:

   a. _____

   b. _____

   c. _____

   d. _____

7. What is one of the early clinical manifestations of prerenal failure?

   Answer: _____

8. List the five categories of renal abnormalities that cause renal failure:

   a. _____

   b. _____

   c. _____

   d. _____

   e. _____

9. List some postrenal abnormalities that cause renal failure:

   a. _____

   b. _____

10. Positive pressure ventilation (_____ increases; _____ decreases) urinary output.

11. Negative pressure ventilation (_____ increases; _____ decreases) urinary output.

12. When positive pressure ventilation causes the blood volume and, therefore, the pressure in the atria to decrease, the release of ADH

   a. increases
   b. decreases
   c. remains the same

13. When the concentration of ADH increases, the amount of urine formed

   a. increases
   b. decreases
   c. remains the same

CARDIOPULMONARY DISORDERS CAUSED BY RENAL FAILURE

1. Hypertension and edema develop in renal failure because of the kidney's inability to excrete

   _____ .

2. When the kidneys fail, metabolic acidosis develops because the following changes occur:

    a. H^+ (_____ increases; _____ decreases)

    b. K^+ (_____ increases; _____ decreases)

    c. HCO_3^- (_____ increases; _____ decreases)

3. Hypochloremia causes (select one)

    a. acidosis
    b. alkalosis

4. Hypokalemia causes (select one)

    a. acidosis
    b. alkalosis

5. Hyperchloremia causes (select one)

    a. acidosis
    b. alkalosis

6. Hyperkalemia causes (select one)

    a. acidosis
    b. alkalosis

7. Which two mechanisms contribute to the anemia seen in chronic renal failure?

    a. _____

    _____

    _____

    _____

    b. _____

    _____

    _____

    _____

8. Why do patients with chronic renal failure have a tendency to bleed?

_____

_____

_____

9. Why is pericarditis seen in about 50 percent of persons with chronic renal failure?

_____

_____

_____

_____

_____

CHAPTER SEVENTEEN

SLEEP PHYSIOLOGY AND ITS RELATIONSHIP TO THE CARDIOPULMONARY SYSTEM

1. Because sleep is readily reversible, it is distinguished from a _____ , which is a state of unconsciousness from which a person cannot be awakened, even by the most forceful stimuli.

2. Body size appears to play an important role in determining the amount of sleep a species needs.

   In general, _____ mammals need less sleep than _____ mammals.

3. A _____ is a polygraphic recording of multiple physiologic variables that is used to identify the different phases of sleep.

4. The major physiologic variables monitored during a sleep study include

   a. _____ , which measures the electrophysiologic changes in the brain;

   b. _____ , which monitors the movements of the eyes; and

   c. _____ which measures muscle activity.

5. Other physiologic features typically monitored during a sleep study include

   a. _____

   b. _____

   c. _____

   d. _____

   e. _____

   f. _____

6. Most sleep study epochs are _____ in duration.

TYPES OF SLEEP

1. _____ and _____

   _____ are the two major types of sleep.

2. The EEG tracing during the eyes open wake state shows _____

   _____ .

3. During the eyes open wake state, the EOG is _____ frequency and variable, and the

   EMG activity is relatively _____ .

4. The EEG during the eyes closed wake (drowsy) period is characterized by prominent

   _____ .

5. The EOG tracing during the eyes closed wake state usually shows _____ .

6. The EMG activity during the eyes closed wake state is relatively _____ .

7. In general, Stages 1 and 2 are described as _____ , and Stages 3 and 4 are referred to

   as _____ sleep stages.

8. Non-REM sleep accounts for about _____ of sleep time in the average adult.

9. In the average young adult, Stage 1 comprises about _____ of sleep time; Stage 2

   about _____ ; and Stage 3 and Stage 4 make up about _____ of total sleep time.

10. **Stage 1** is the _____ stage between drowsiness and sleep.

11. The sleeper frequently experiences sudden muscle contractions called _____ .

12. As the patient moves into Stage 1, the EEG shows light sleep comprised of _____

    _____ . Some _____ may also appear.

13. _____ commonly appear toward the end of Stage 1. The EOG shows _____

    movements. The EMG reveals _____ .

14. **Stage 2** is still a relatively _____ .

15. In Stage 2, the EEG becomes more _____ and is comprised predominantly of _____,

    intermixed with sudden bursts of _____, and one or more _____.

    _____ may also be seen during this stage.

16. In Stage 2, the EOG shows either _____ eye movements or _____ eye movements.

17. In Stage 2, the EMG has _____ electrical activity.

18. In Stage 2, the heart rate, blood pressure, respiratory rate, and temperature _____ slightly.

19. Stage 2 occupies the greatest proportion of the total sleep time and accounts for about

    _____ of sleep.

20. **Stage 3** (medium deep sleep) is present when _____ of the EEG activity consists of

    _____, slow _____.

21. Both _____ and _____ may be present during Stage 3.

22. In Stage 3, there is _____ on the EOG, and the EMG activity is _____.

23. **Stage 4** (deep slow-wave sleep) is present when more than _____ of the EEG activity

    consists of _____.

24. In Stage 4, the EOG shows ___ eye movements, and the EMG has _____ electrical activity.

25. In Stage 4, the sleeper's heart and respiratory rate generally decrease _____ percent below
    the person's normal waking hour levels.

26. REM sleep resembles the _____.

27. In REM sleep, the EEG reveals _____, and frequent _____.

    _____ may be present.

28. In REM sleep, the EOG shows _____.

29. In REM sleep, the EMG recording shows _____, and a temporary

    _____ of most of the skeletal muscles (e.g., arms, legs) is present.

30. In REM sleep, the breathing rate _____ and _____ irregularly.

31. The heart rate during REM sleep becomes inconsistent with episodes of _____ and _____ rates.

32. About _____ percent of the sleep of the young normal adult consists of REM sleep.

33. The first REM sleep period usually occurs about _____ minutes after one falls asleep, and lasts _____ minutes.

34. REM is not as _____ as NREM sleep. In fact, REM sleep is also known as _____ , since the EEG pattern is similar to the normal awake pattern.

35. Most _____ occur during REM sleep. They are frequently remembered during the wakeful state, and are often described as having _____ _____ .

NORMAL SLEEP CYCLES

1. Under normal circumstances, most people require _____ minutes to fall asleep.

2. The time needed to fall asleep is called _____ .

3. A sleep latency period less than _____ minutes indicates _____ sleepiness.

4. A sleep latency period longer than _____ minutes is associated with _____ _____ .

5. One full sleep cycle begins with Stage _____ . The sleeper then progresses through Stages _____ ; followed by a return to Stages _____ . From Stage _____ , the sleeper slips into _____ sleep. The end of REM sleep is the conclusion of the _____ .

6. From REM sleep, the individual moves back to Stage _____ and a new _____ begins.

7. The duration of each sleep cycle is about _____ minutes.

8. The sleep cycles become _____ as the sleeper becomes rested.

9. Between _____ full cycles of sleep occur during a normal night's sleep.

10. The normal young adult moves from Stages 1 to 4 in about _____ minutes.

11. The sleeper usually remains in Stage 4 for about _____ minutes.

12. The first REM sleep lasts for about _____ minutes.

13. As the night progresses, REM sleep periods _____ in duration and deep sleep (Stages 3 and 4) _____ .

14. If awakened during any stage, the sleeper must return to Stage _____ sleep and proceed through all the stages.

15. By morning, the majority of sleep is spent in _____ .

16. Older sleeping adults, in either Stage 2 or 3 NREM sleep, often bypass _____ sleep altogether and awaken.

17. Except for the older adult, changes in body position during sleep usually occur _____ times during the night.

18. One or two _____ are normal for the young adult.

19. The number and duration of awakenings tend to _____ with age.

FUNCTIONS OF SLEEP

1. The two most widely accepted theories regarding the purpose of sleep are _____ and

   _____ .

2. The most widely accepted theory of sleep function is that it provides the body with a period for

   _____ and _____ .

3. It is thought that non-REM, slow-wave sleep promotes _____ and _____ . This theory is further supported by the fact that slow-wave sleep coincides with the release of

   _____ in children and young adults.

4. Many of the body's cells also show _____ production and reduced breakdown of

   _____ during deep sleep.

5. REM sleep appears to play an important role in the restoration of the brain processes, such as

   _____ .

6. Some suggest that sleep is an extension of _____ .

7. The metabolic rate decreases _____ during non-REM slow-wave sleep.

8. The conservation theory is further supported by the fact that slow-wave sleep _____ with age.

CIRCADIAN RHYTHMS

1. **Biologic rhythms** that occur at regular intervals of about 24 hours are called _____ .

2. Examples of biorhythms include the

   a. _____

   b. _____

   c. _____

3. When an individual's biologic clock corresponds to a good sleep–wake pattern, the person is said

   to be in _____ .

4. Current publications involving sleep, sleep deprivation, and sleep disorders strongly suggest that

   the number-one sleep-related problem affecting most people today is _____ .

NORMAL SLEEP PATTERNS

1. Sleep patterns are well established in the first _____ of life and continue throughout life.

2. With advancing age, regular sleep patterns gradually _____ .

3. The **newborn** sleeps about _____ hours a day. However, this total sleep time is usually

   divided into about _____ fairly equal sleep periods throughout the day and night.

4. Initially, the infant usually awakens every ____ or ____ hours, eats, and then goes back to sleep.

5. About 50 percent of the sleep period is spent in _____ , and about 50 percent is spent

   in _____ .

6. During the REM periods, the infant commonly exhibits a lot of _____ , such as

   _____ .

7. By ____ months, most infants sleep through the night and take short naps throughout the day.

8. At the end of one year, most infants sleep about ____ hours a day and take one or two naps during daylight hours.

9. In regard to **toddlers** and **preschoolers**, the total sleep time declines from about 14 hours a day at age ____ to about 12 hours a day by the _____ year.

10. School-age children sleep between ____ and ____ hours a day.

11. Most **adolescents** need between ____ and ____ hours of sleep.

12. The **young adult** usually requires between ____ and ____ hours of sleep a day.

13. In the young adult, Stages 3 and 4 progressively _____ , and the number of arousals from sleep _____ .

14. The **older adult** needs about ____ hours of sleep a day.

15. In the older adult, Stages 3 and 4 are significantly _____ .

16. Older adults frequently require _____ periods of time to fall asleep.

FACTORS AFFECTING SLEEP

1. List common factors that affect sleep.

   a. _____

   b. _____

   c. _____

   d. _____

   e. _____

   f. _____

   g. _____

   h. _____

   i. _____

   j. _____

   k. _____

COMMON SLEEP DISORDERS

1. List common sleep disorders.

    a. _____

    b. _____

    c. _____

    d. _____

    e. _____

    f. _____

NORMAL CARDIOPULMONARY PHYSIOLOGY DURING SLEEP

1. In general, at sleep onset there is an increased parasympathetic activity, which continues throughout non-REM sleep. The parasympathetic tone continues to increase during the transition to REM sleep. This increased parasympathetic activity causes a number of autonomic nervous system changes throughout which areas of the body?

    a. _____

    b. _____

    c. _____

    d. _____

    e. _____

    f. _____

    g. _____

    h. _____

    i. _____

    j. _____

2. During REM sleep, neural impulses to most skeletal muscles stop and a lack of muscle tone ensues. In essence, the sleeper is temporarily _____ .

   _____ .

3. In severe cases, this condition can lead to _____ .

   _____ .

4. The body temperature usually falls by ____ to ____ Celsius during non-REM sleep.

5. Renal perfusion is _____ during non-REM sleep, resulting in _____ urine production.

6. During sleep, salivation and esophageal motility (swallowing) are markedly _____ .

7. During sleep there is also a _____ colonic function, which, in turn, results in a _____ colonic motility.

8. When the sleeper awakens in the morning, the colonic motility _____ significantly.

9. Patients with obstructive sleep apnea or narcolepsy commonly have a _____ correlation between sleep and growth hormone concentration.

10. The heart rate variations during non-REM sleep follow a _____ pattern.

11. During REM sleep, the heart rate becomes inconsistent, with episodes of _____ and _____ rates.

12. The increased activity of the vagal nerve during non-REM sleep results in decreased _____ , _____ , and _____ .

13. On the other hand, the surge of autonomic activity during REM sleep increases the _____ and increases the risk for _____ .

14. During non-REM sleep, there is a _____ in cerebral blood flow.

15. During REM sleep, there is an _____ in cerebral blood flow.

16. In non-REM sleep, the respiratory rate _____ .

17. During REM sleep, however, the respiratory rate _____ and _____ irregularly.

Section III
THE CARDIOPULMONARY SYSTEM DURING UNUSUAL ENVIRONMENTAL CONDITIONS

CHAPTER EIGHTEEN

EXERCISE AND ITS EFFECTS ON THE CARDIOPULMONARY SYSTEM

EFFECTS OF EXERCISE

1. During heavy exercise

    a. Alveolar ventilation may increase as much as _____-fold.

    b. Oxygen diffusion capacity may increase as much as _____-fold.

    c. Cardiac output may increase as much as _____-fold.

    d. Muscle blood flow may increase as much as _____-fold.

    e. Oxygen consumption may increase as much as _____-fold.

    f. Heat production may increase as much as _____-fold.

2. Muscle training can increase muscle size and strength _____ to _____ percent.

3. The efficiency of intracellular metabolism may increase by _____ to _____ percent.

4. The size of the heart chambers and the heart mass of well-trained athletes may be increased by _____ percent.

5. The point at which anaerobic metabolism develops is called the _____ .

VENTILATION

1. It has been suggested that the increased ventilation seen in exercise is caused by

   a. _____

   _____

   _____

   b. _____

   _____

   _____

   c. _____

   _____

   _____

2. During strenuous exercise, an adult alveolar ventilation can increase to

   a. 40 L/min
   b. 60 L/min
   c. 80 L/min
   d. 100 L/min
   e. 120 L/min

3. During exercise, the increased alveolar ventilation is caused mainly by an increased _____ of ventilation, rather than by an increased _____ of ventilation.

4. During very heavy exercise, both an increased _____ and _____ of ventilation are seen.

5. During very heavy exercise, the tidal volume is usually about what percent (circle one) of the vital capacity?

   a. 10 percent
   b. 20 percent
   c. 30 percent
   d. 40 percent
   e. 50 percent
   f. 60 percent

6. There are three distinct consecutive breathing patterns seen during mild and moderate exercise.

   a. The **first stage** is characterized by _____

_____

_____

_____

   b. The **second stage** is typified by _____

_____

_____

_____

   c. During the **third stage,** _____

_____

7. The maximum alveolar ventilation generated during heavy exercise under normal conditions is

about _____ to _____ percent of the maximum voluntary ventilation.

8. At rest, normal oxygen consumption ($\dot{V}_{O_2}$) is about _____ mL per minute.

9. During exercise, the skeletal muscles may account for more than _____ percent of the $\dot{V}_{O_2}$.

10. The Pa_{O_2} remains constant during
    I. mild exercise
   II. moderate exercise
  III. heavy exercise

    a. I only
    b. I and II only
    c. I, II, and III

11. It has been shown that the increased oxygen diffusion capacity results from the _____

_____ during exercise.

12. During exercise, the $P_{(A-a)O_2}$ remains essentially constant until what percent (circle one) of the maximal oxygen consumption is reached?

    a. 10 percent
    b. 20 percent
    c. 30 percent
    d. 40 percent
    e. 50 percent

CIRCULATION

1. During exercise these essential physiologic responses must occur in order for the circulatory system to supply the working muscles with an adequate amount of blood:

    a. _____

    b. _____

    c. _____

2. The two circulatory effects of a sympathetic discharge are that

    a. _____

    _____

    _____

    _____

    b. _____

    _____

    _____

    _____

3. The increased oxygen demands during exercise are met almost entirely by _____

    _____ .

4. The increased cardiac output during exercise results from

   a. _____

   b. _____

   c. _____

5. The increased stroke volume during exercise is primarily caused by _____ in the working muscles.

6. The ability of the heart to accommodate the increased venous return and, subsequently, increase cardiac output is due to the _____ curve.

7. The maximum heart rate for a 55-year-old person is about _____ .

8. When the stroke volume decreases, the heart rate (_____ increases; _____ decreases; _____ remains the same), and when the stroke volume increases, the heart rate (_____ increases; _____ decreases; _____ remains the same).

9. The stroke volume is influenced by

   a. _____

   _____

   b. _____

   _____

   c. _____

   _____

10. The body's ability to increase the heart rate and stroke volume during exercise progressively (_____ increases; _____ decreases) with age.

11. There is an increase in arterial blood pressure during exercise because of

   a. _____

   _____

   _____

   b. _____

   _____

   _____

   c. _____

   _____

   _____

12. As oxygen consumption and cardiac output increase during exercise, the pulmonary

   a. systolic pressure (_____ increases; _____ decreases; _____ remains the same)

   b. diastolic pressure (_____ increases; _____ decreases; _____ remains the same)

   c. arterial (mean) pressure (_____ increases; _____ decreases; _____ remains the same)

   d. wedge pressure (_____ increases; _____ decreases; _____ remains the same)

13. The dilation of the blood vessels in the working muscles is caused primarily by _____

   _____ acting on the arterioles.

STROKE VOLUME VERSUS HEART RATE IN INCREASING CARDIAC OUTPUT

1. During very heavy exercise, the increased _____ accounts for a much greater proportion of the increased cardiac output than the _____ .

2. The stroke volume reaches its maximum when the maximum cardiac output is only at approximately _____ percent.

3. After the stroke volume reaches its maximum, any further increase in cardiac output is solely

   caused by an _____ .

4. Maximum exercise taxes the respiratory system only about _____ percent of maximum.

BODY TEMPERATURE/CUTANEOUS BLOOD FLOW RELATIONSHIP

1. List the symptoms that, collectively, are referred to as heat stroke:

   _____

   _____

   _____

   _____

   _____

   _____

2. The primary treatment of heat stroke consists of

   a. _____

   _____

   b. _____

   _____

   c. _____

   _____

   d. _____

   _____

CARDIOPULMINARY REHABILITATION

1. List the three phase(s) of the **cardiopulminary rehabilitation** process:

   a. Phase I: _____

   _____

   b. Phase II: _____

   _____

   _____

   c. Phase III: _____

   _____

CHAPTER NINETEEN

HIGH ALTITUDE AND ITS EFFECTS ON THE CARDIOPULMONARY SYSTEM

HIGH ALTITUDE

1. The barometric pressure is about half the sea level value of 760 mm Hg at an altitude of

   _____ feet.

2. One of the most prominent features of acclimatization is _____

   _____

3. In lowlanders who ascend to high altitudes, the RBCs increase for about _____ before the production rate levels off.

4. People who live at high altitudes commonly demonstrate

   a. mild respiratory acidosis
   b. normal arterial blood gas values
   c. mild respiratory alkalosis

5. The oxygen diffusion capacity of lowlanders who are acclimatized to high altitude

   a. increases
   b. decreases
   c. remains the same

6. The oxygen diffusion capacity of high-altitude natives is about _____ than predicted.

7. At high altitude, the alveolar-arterial P_{O_2} difference [$P_{(A-a)O_2}$]

   a. increases
   b. decreases
   c. remains the same

8. At high altitude, the overall ventilation-perfusion ratio improves in response to the (_____

   increased; _____ decreased) pulmonary arterial blood pressure.

9. In individuals who have acclimatized to high altitude, and in high-altitude natives, cardiac output

   a. increases
   b. decreases
   c. remains the same

10. As an individual ascends, the pulmonary vascular system

   a. constricts
   b. dilates
   c. remains the same

OTHER PHYSIOLOGIC CHANGES

1. In high-altitude natives, the concentration of myoglobin in skeletal muscles

   a. increases
   b. decreases
   c. remains the same

2. **Acute mountain sickness** is characterized by _____

   _____

   _____

   _____

3. The symptoms of acute mountain sickness are generally most severe on the _____

   _____

   _____

4. Although the exact cause of high-altitude pulmonary edema is not fully understood, it may be

   associated with pulmonary (_____ vasoconstriction; _____ vasodilation), and with a/an (_____

   increased; _____ decreased) permeability of the pulmonary capillaries.

5. High-altitude cerebral edema is characterized by_____

_____

_____

_____

6. **Chronic mountain sickness** is characterized by_____

_____

_____

_____

CHAPTER TWENTY

HIGH-PRESSURE ENVIRONMENTS AND THEIR EFFECTS ON THE CARDIOPULMONARY SYSTEM

DIVING

1. For every 33 feet below the water surface, the pressure increases _____ .

2. a. If an individual fully inhales to a total lung capacity of 5.5 liters at sea level, and dives to a depth of 99 feet, the lungs will be compressed to about

   Answer: _____

   b. What is the pressure within the above diver's lungs?

   Answer: _____

3. The maximum time of a breath-hold dive is a function of

   a. _____

   _____

   b. _____

   _____

4. In regard to the P_{CO_2}, the so-called respiratory drive **breaking point** is about _____ mm Hg.

5. The so-called CO_2 paradox occurs as a diver (_____ descends; _____ ascends) and the O_2 paradox

   occurs as the diver (_____ descends; _____ ascends).

6. The fall in $P_{A_{O_2}}$ as a diver returns to the surface is known as the _____

   _____ .

7. The **mammalian diving reflex** consists of

   a. _____

   b. _____

   c. _____

   d. _____

8. List some of the signs and symptoms collectively referred to as **decompression sickness**:

   a. _____

   b. _____

   c. _____

   d. _____

   e. _____

HYPERBARIC MEDICINE

1. Identify indications for hyperbaric oxygenation for the following clinical conditions:

TABLE 20–1 Indications for Hyperbaric Oxygenation

Gas Diseases

Vascular Insufficiency States

Infections

Defects in Oxygen Transport

---

2. Hyperbaric oxygen is effective in the treatment of carbon monoxide poisoning. The administration of hyperbaric oxygen

   a. _____

   _____

   _____

   _____

   b. _____

   _____

   _____

   _____

   c. _____

   _____

   _____

   _____

3. Breathing 100 percent oxygen at one atmosphere changes the CO_{Hb} half-life to less than _____

   _____ .

ANSWERS TO CHAPTER EXERCISES

The question numbers refer to the questions in this workbook. For any problem areas, refer back to the appropriate section in the textbook, *Cardiopulmonary Anatomy and Physiology: Essentials for Respiratory Care*, Fifth edition.

CHAPTER ONE

THE ANATOMY AND PHYSIOLOGY OF THE RESPIRATORY SYSTEM

THE UPPER AIRWAY

1. (Fig. 1-1, pg. 8)
2. a. to act as a conductor of air
   b. to humidity and warm the inspired air
   c. to prevent foreign materials from entering the tracheobronchial tree
   d. to serve as an important area involved in speech and smell
3. a. filter
   b. humidify
   c. warm
4. (Fig. 1-2, pg. 8)
5. (Fig. 1-3, pg. 9)
6. pseudostratified ciliated columnar
7. a. superior nasal turbinate
   b. middle nasal turbinate
   c. inferior nasal turbinate
8. (Fig. 1-5, pg. 11)
9. levator veli palatinum
10. stratified squamous
11. palatoglossal, palatopharyngeal
12. pseudostratified ciliated columnar
13. eustachian tube
14. stratified squamous
15. stratified squamous
16. (Fig. 1-6, pg. 12)
17. a. acts as a passageway of air between the pharynx and the trachea
    b. works as a protective mechanism against the aspiration of solids and liquids
    c. generates sounds for speech
18. (Fig. 1-7, pg. 14)
19. (Fig. 1-11, pg. 18)
20. vocal ligament
21. thyroid cartilage
22. rima glottidis or glottis
23. stratified squamous
24. pseudostratified ciliated columnar
25. Valsalva's maneuver
26. (Fig. 1-13, pg. 21)
27. (Fig. 1-14, pg. 22)

THE LOWER AIRWAYS

1. (Fig. 1-15, pg. 23)
2. a. epithelial lining
   b. lamina propria
   c. cartilaginous layer
3. pseudostratified ciliated columnar
4. submucosal glands
5. sol layer, gel layer
6. (Fig. 1-17, pg. 26)
7. a. cigarette smoke
   b. dehydration
   c. positive pressure ventilation
   d. endotracheal suctioning
   e. high inspired oxygen concentrations
   f. hypoxia
   g. atmospheric pollutants
   h. general anesthetics
   i. parasympatholytics
8. a. histamine
   b. heparin
   c. slow-reacting substance of anaphylaxis
   d. platelet-activating factor
   e. eosinophilic chemotactic factor of anaphylaxis
   f. leukotrienes
9. 11 to 13, 1.5 to 2.5
10. carina
11. 25, 40 to 60
12. terminal bronchioles
13. increases
14. terminal bronchioles
15. mediastinal lymph nodes, the pulmonary nerves, a portion of the esophagus, and the visceral pleura
16. azygos, hemiazygos, intercostal veins
17. bronchopulmonary anastomoses

THE SITES OF GAS EXCHANGE

1. a. respiratory
   b. alveolar
   c. alveolar
2. (Fig. 1-25, pg. 36)
3. (Fig. 1-26, pg. 37)
4. 300
5. 70
6. respiratory bronchioles, alveolar ducts, and alveolar clusters

7. 130,000
8. a. acinus
   b. terminal respiratory unit
   c. lung parenchyma
   d. functional units
9. squamous pneumocyte
10. granular pneumocyte
11. 95
12. type II
13. pores of Kohn
14. alveolar macrophages
15. tight space, loose space

PULMONARY VASCULAR SYSTEM AND LYMPHATIC SYSTEM

1. (Fig. 1-29, pg. 41)
2. resistance
3. 0.1 μm, 10 μm
4. capacitance
5. visceral pleura
6. loose space of the interstitium
7. (Fig. 1-31, pg. 45)

NEURAL CONTROL OF THE LUNGS

1. autonomic nervous system
3. epinephrine or norepinephrine
4. relax
5. constrict
6. acetylcholine

THE LUNGS

1. first
2. sixth, eleventh
3. hilum
4. costal, mediastinal
5. oblique fissure, fourth
6. costal, mediastinal
7. (Fig. 1-33, pg. 47)
8. (Fig. 1-34, pg. 47)
9. (Fig. 1-36, pg. 49)
10. (Fig. 1-37, pg. 50)

THE MEDIASTINUM, PLEURAL MEMBRANES, AND THORAX

1. trachea, heart, major blood vessels, various nerves, portions of the esophagus, thymus gland, and lymph nodes
2. visceral
3. parietal
4. pleural cavity
5. a. manubrium sterni
   b. the body
   c. xiphoid process
6. true ribs
7. false
8. floating
9. (Fig. 1-38, pg. 51)
10. (Fig. 1-39, pg. 52)

THE DIAPHRAGM

1. central tendon
2. esophagus, aorta, several nerves, and inferior vena cava
3. phrenic
4. first, second
5. sternum
6. chest, anteroposterior
7. scapula, shoulders, arms
8. upward, outward
9. (Fig. 1-48, pg. 59)
10. downward, inward

CHAPTER TWO

VENTILATION

PRESSURE DIFFERENCES ACROSS THE LUNGS

1. driving pressure
2. transairway pressure
3. positive transmural pressure
4. negative transmural pressure
5. transpulmonary pressure
6. transthoracic pressure
7. 5 mm Hg
8. 7 mm Hg
9. 4 mm Hg
10. 6 mm Hg
11. decrease
12. greater
13. below
14. 3 to 6, 2 to 4

ELASTIC PROPERTIES OF THE LUNG AND CHEST WALL

1. volume, pressure

Case A

2. a. 0.055 L/cm H_2O (55 ml/cm H_2O)
   b. 0.070 L/cm H_2O (70 ml/cm H_2O)
   c. increasing

Case B

3. a. 0.050 L/cm H_2O (50 ml/cm H_2O)
   b. 0.045 L/cm H_2O (45 ml/cm H_2O)
   c. decreasing
4. 0.1 L/cm H_2O
5. 2,000 ml (2 liters)
6. right
7. a
8. b
9. the natural ability of matter to respond directly to force and to return to its original resting position or shape after the external force no longer exists

10. the change in pressure per change in volume

$$\text{Elastance} = \frac{\Delta P}{\Delta V}$$

11. low, high
12. when a truly elastic body, like a spring, is acted on by 1 unit of force, the elastic body will stretch 1 unit of length, and when acted on by 2 units of force it will stretch 2 units of length, and so forth
13. volume, pressure
14. surface tension
15. 70 dynes/cm

16. $P = \dfrac{2ST}{r}$

17. a. directly proportional to the surface tension of the liquid
    b. inversely proportional to the radius of the sphere
18. increases, decreases
19. b
20. critical opening pressure
21. c
22. alveolar type II cells
23. water insoluble, water soluble
24. increases, decrease
25. 5–15 dynes, 50 dynes
26. a. acidosis
    b hypoxia
    c. hyperoxia
    d. atelectasis
    e. pulmonary vascular congestion
27. low

DYNAMIC CHARACTERISTICS OF THE LUNGS

1. study of forces in action
2. the movement in action of gas in and out of the lungs and the pressure changes required to move the gas

3. $\dot{V} = \dfrac{\Delta P r^4 \pi}{8 l \eta}$

4. a. increases
   b. increases
   c. increases
   d. increases

5. a. 2 liters/minute (L/min)
   b. 14 L/min
   c. 256 cm H_2O
   d. 20 cm H_2O
   e. 10 L/min
   f. 50 L/min
   g. 160 cm H_2O
   h. 10 cm H_2O

6. $\dot{V} = Pr^4$

   $$P = \frac{\dot{V}}{r^4}$$

AIRWAY RESISTANCE AND DYNAMIC COMPLIANCE

1. pressure difference between the mouth and the alveoli divided by flow rate

2. $R_{aw} = \dfrac{\Delta P(cm\ H_2O)}{\dot{V}(L/sec)}$

3. 3 cm H_2O/L/sec
4. 0.5, 1.5
5. a gas flow that is streamlined
6. molecules that move through a tube in a random manner
7. time (in seconds) necessary to inflate a particular lung region to about 60 percent of its potential filling capacity
8. b
9. b
10. c
11. a
12. a
13. e
14. change in the volume of the lungs divided by the change in the transpulmonary pressure during the time required for one breath
15. equal to
16. decreases
17. alveoli distal to an obstruction that do not have enough time to fill to their potential filling capacity as the breathing frequency increases

VENTILATORY PATTERNS

1. a. tidal volume
   b. ventilatory rate
   c. time relationship between inhalation and exhalation
2. 7 to 9, 3 to 4
3. 15

4. 1 : 2
5. alveolar ventilation
6. dead space ventilation
7. the volume of gas in the conducting airways: the nose, mouth, pharynx, larynx, and lower airways down to, but not including, the respiratory bronchioles
8. 130 mL
9. tidal volume, dead space ventilation, breaths per minute
10. 6,240 mL
11. an alveolus that is ventilated but not perfused with pulmonary blood
12. the sum of the anatomic dead space and alveolar dead space
13. greater
14. larger
15. c
16. increases, decreases
17. decreases, increases
18. energy, ventilation
19. complete absence of spontaneous ventilation
20. normal, spontaneous breathing
21. short episodes of rapid, uniformly deep inspirations, followed by 10 to 30 seconds of apnea
22. increased depth of breathing with or without an increased frequency
23. an increased alveolar ventilation produced by any ventilatory pattern that causes the $P_{A_{CO_2}}$ and, therefore, the Pa_{CO_2} to decrease
24. a decreased alveolar ventilation produced by any ventilatory pattern that causes the $P_{A_{CO_2}}$ and, therefore, the Pa_{CO_2} to increase
25. a rapid breathing rate
26. 10 to 30 seconds of apnea, followed by a gradual increase in the volume and frequency of breathing, followed by a gradual decrease in the volume of breathing until another period of apnea occurs
27. both an increased depth and rate of breathing
28. a condition in which an individual is able to breathe most comfortably in the upright position
29. difficulty in breathing, of which the individual is consciously aware

CHAPTER THREE

THE DIFFUSION OF PULMONARY GASES

DIFFUSION AND GAS LAWS

1. the movement of gas molecules from an area of relatively high concentration of gas to one of low concentration
2. if temperature remains constant, pressure will vary inversely to volume
3. $P_1 \times V_1 = P_2 \times V_2$
4. 66.66 cm H_2O
5. 37.5 cm H_2O
6. if pressure remains constant, volume and temperature will vary directly
7. $V_1/T_1 = V_2/T_2$
8. 9.37 L
9. 4.64 L
10. if the volume remains constant, pressure and temperature will vary directly
11. $P_1/T_1 = P_2/T_2$
12. 156.2 cm H_2O
13. 44.53 cm H_2O
14. in a mixture of gases, the total pressure is equal to the sum of the partial pressures of each separate gas
15. 650 mm Hg

THE PARTIAL PRESSURES OF ATMOSPHERIC GASES

2. decreases, remains the same
4. the alveolar oxygen must mix—or compete, in terms of partial pressures—with alveolar CO_2 pressure and alveolar water vapor pressure
5. 44 mg/L, 47 mm Hg
6. 428.2 mm Hg

THE DIFFUSION OF PULMONARY GASES

1. a. liquid lining the intra-alveolar membrane
   b. alveolar epithelial cell
   c. basement membrane of the alveolar epithelial cell
   d. loose connective tissue (the interstitial space)
   e. basement membrane of the capillary endothelium
   f. capillary endothelium
   g. plasma in the capillary blood
   h. erythrocyte membrane
   i. intracellular fluid in the erythrocyte
2. 0.36 and 2.5 μm
3. 40, 46
4. 60, 6
5. 0.25
6. 0.75, one-third
7. b
8. $\dot{V}$ gas L $\dfrac{AD(P_1 - P_2)}{T}$

9. a. a
   b. a
   c. b
10. the amount of gas that dissolves in a liquid at a given temperature is proportional to the partial pressure of the gas
11. solubility coefficient
12. a. directly proportional to the solubility coefficient of the gas
    b. inversely proportional to the square root of the gram-molecular weight of the gas

PERFUSION- AND DIFFUSION-LIMITED GAS FLOW

1. the transfer of gas across the alveolar wall is a function of the amount of blood that flows past the alveoli
2. the movement of gas across the alveolar wall is a function of the integrity of the alveolar-capillary membrane itself
3. a

CHAPTER FOUR

PULMONARY FUNCTION MEASUREMENTS

LUNG VOLUMES AND CAPACITIES

1. the volume of air that normally moves into and out of the lungs in one quiet breath.
2. the maximum volume of air that can be inhaled after a normal tidal volume inhalation.
3. the maximum volume of air that can be exhaled after a normal tidal volume exhalation.
4. the amount of air remaining in the lungs after a maximal exhalation.
5. the maximum volume of air that can be exhaled after a maximal inspiration.
6. the volume of air that can be inhaled after a normal exhalation.
7. the volume of air remaining in the lungs after a normal exhalation.
8. maximum amount of air that the lungs can accommodate.
9. the percentage of the TLC occupied by the RV.
11. RV, V_T, FRC, RV/TLC ratio; VC, IC, IRV, ERV
12. VC, IC, RV, FRC, V_T, TLC
13. a. closed circuit helium dilution
    b. open circuit nitrogen washout
    c. body plethysmography

PULMONARY MECHANICS

1. the maximum volume of gas that can be exhaled as forcefully and rapidly as possible after a maximal inspiration.
2. the maximum volume of gas that can be exhaled within a specific period of time.
3. a. 60
   b. 83
   c. 94
   d. 97
4. decreases
5. comparison of the amount of air exhaled in 1 second to the total amount exhaled during a FVC maneuver.
6. forced expiratory volume in 1 second percentage ($FEV_{1\%}$).
7. 83 percent
8. a. determine the severity of a patient's obstructive pulmonary disease
   b. distinguish between an obstructive and restrictive lung disorder

238

9. decreased
10. normal or increased
11. the average flow rate during the middle 50 percent of an FVC measurement.
12. medium, small
13. the average rate of airflow between 200 and 1,200 mL of the FVC.
14. large
15. the maximum flow rate that can be achieved during an FVC manuever.
16. the largest volume of gas that can be breathed voluntarily in and out of the lungs in 1 minute.
17. (Fig. 4-12, pg. 166)

EFFECTS OF DYNAMIC COMPRESSION ON EXPIRATORY FLOW RATES

1. dependent on the amount of muscular effort exerted by the individual.
2. effort-dependent
3. once a maximum flow rate has been attained, the flow rate cannot be increased by further muscular effort.
4. dynamic compression
5. toward the alveolus (upstream)
6. increases

CHAPTER FIVE

THE ANATOMY AND PHYSIOLOGY OF THE CIRCULATORY SYSTEM

THE BLOOD

1. a. plasma
   b. erythrocytes
   c. leukocytes
   d. thrombocytes
2. erythrocytes
3. 5
4. 4
5. hematocrit
6. a. 45
   b. 42
   c. 45, 60
7. 7.5 μm, 2.5 μm
8. 120
9. protect the body against the invasion of bacteria, viruses, parasites, toxins, and tumors.
10. 4000 to 11,000
12. neutrophils
13. eosinophils
14. lymphocytes
15. Lymphocytes
16. platelets
17. 250,000 and 500,000
18. prevent blood loss from a traumatized surface of the body involving the smallest blood vessels.
19. 55
20. 90
21. a. albumins
    b. globulins
    c. fibrinogen
22. a. Na^+
    b. K^+
    c. Ca^{2+}
    d. Mg^{2+}

23. a. Cl^-
    b. PO_4^{3-}
    c. SO_4^{2-}
    d. HCO_3^-
24. a. amino acids
    b. glucose/carbohydrates
    c. lipids
    d. individual vitamins
25. a. urea
    b. creatinine
    c. uric acid
    d. bilirubin

THE HEART

1. (Fig. 5-2, pg. 189)
2. atria, ventricles
3. interatrial septum, interventricular septum
4. unoxygenated blood to the lungs
5. oxygenated blood throughout the systemic circulation
6. 250, 350
7. point of maximal intensity (PMI)

The Pericardium

1. pericardium
2. a. protect the heart.
   b. anchor it to surrounding structures, such as the diaphragm and the great vessels.
   c. prevent the heart from overfilling.
3. parietal layer, visceral layer

The Wall of the Heart

1. a single sheet of squamous epithelial cells overlying delicate connective tissue
2. cross-striated tissue fibers that form a network of spiral bundles throughout the internal portion of the heart
3. inner myocardial surface; it lines the heart chambers

Blood Supply of the Heart

1. left coronary artery, the right coronary artery
2. circumflex, anterior interventricular branches
3. marginal branch, posterior interventricular branch
4. great cardiac veins
5. middle cardiac vein
6. coronary sinus
7. thebesian veins

Blood Flow through the Heart

1. inferior and superior vena cava
2. thebesian veins
3. tricuspid valve
4. chordae tendinae
5. papillary muscles
6. pulmonary trunk, pulmonary arteries
7. pulmonary semilunar valve
8. pulmonary veins
9. bicuspid valve (also called the mitral valve)
10. aorta

THE PULMONARY AND SYSTEMIC VASCULAR SYSTEMS

1. pulmonary trunk, left atrium
2. aorta, right atrium
3. away from
4. arterioles
5. arterioles
6. arterioles
7. external
8. internal
9. venules
10. capacitance
11. 60
12. sympathetic
13. vasomotor, medulla oblongata, sympathetic
14. sympathetic
15. vasomotor tone
16. increasing, sympathetic
17. decreasing, sympathetic
18. a. heart
    b. brain
    c. skeletal muscles

19. pressoreceptors
20. glossopharyngeal
21. vagus
22. decrease, increase
23. a. an increased cardiac output
    b. an increase in the total peripheral resistance
    c. the return of blood pressure toward normal
24. a. large arteries
    b. large veins
    c. pulmonary vessels
    d. cardiac walls

PRESSURES IN THE PULMONARY AND SYSTEMIC VASCULAR SYSTEMS

1. actual blood pressure in the lumen of any vessel at any point, relative to the barometric pressure.
2. difference between the pressure in the lumen of a vessel and the pressure surrounding the vessel.
3. greater than
4. less than
5. difference between the pressure at one point in a vessel and the pressure at any other point downstream in the vessel.

THE CARDIAC CYCLE AND ITS EFFECT ON BLOOD PRESSURE

1. systolic pressure
2. diastolic pressure
3. 125 mm Hg
4. 10
5. (Fig. 5-14, pg. 204)
6. 40, 80 mL
7. cardiac output
8. 4,400 mL/min
9. a
10. 5
11. 75, 15, 10
12. 60, 10

THE DISTRIBUTION OF PULMONARY BLOOD FLOW

1. to the portion of the body, or portion of the organ, that is closest to the ground.
2. greater than
3. a. posterior
   b. anterior
   c. lateral half of the lung nearest the ground
   d. apices
4. greater than
5. a. severe hemorrhage
   b. dehydration
   c. positive pressure ventilation
6. alveolar dead space
7. greater than, greater than
8. greater than, less than
9. a. ventricular preload
   b. ventricular afterload
   c. myocardial contractility
10. the degree to which the myocardial fiber is stretched prior to contraction.
11. more
12. ventricular end-diastolic pressure
13. ventricular end-diastolic volume
14. a
15. Frank-Starling curve
16. the force against which the ventricles must work to pump blood.
17. a. the volume and viscosity of blood ejected
    b. peripheral vascular resistance
    c. total cross-sectional area of the vascular space into which blood is ejected
18. arterial systolic blood pressure
19. $BP = CO \times SVR$
20. the force generated by the myocardium when the ventricular muscle fibers shorten.
21. b
22. a. pulse
    b. blood pressure
    c. skin temperature
    d. serial hemodynamic measurements
23. positive inotropism
24. negative inotropism

25. $\text{Resistance} = \dfrac{\text{mean arterial pressure}}{\text{cardiac output}}$

26. a

Active Mechanisms Affecting Vascular Resistance

1. the physiologic, pharmacologic, or pathologic processes that have a direct effect on the vascular system
2. a
3. a
4. a
5. a
6. a. epinephrine (Adrenaline)
   b. norepinephrine (Levophed)
   c. dobutamine (Dobutrex)
   d. dopamine (Intropin)
   e. phenylephrine (Neo-synephrine)
7. a. oxygen
   b. isoproterenol (Isuprel)
   c. aminophylline
   d. calcium-channel blocking agents
8. a. vessel blockage or obstruction
   b. vessel wall diseases
   c. vessel destruction or obliteration
   d. vessel compression

Passive Mechanisms Affecting Vascular Resistance

1. a secondary change in pulmonary vascular resistance that occurs in response to another mechanical change
2. b
3. the opening of vessels that were closed, the stretching or widening of vessels that were open.
4. b
5. high
6. low
7. low
8. high
9. low
10. high
11. b
12. a

CHAPTER SIX

OXYGEN TRANSPORT

OXYGEN TRANSPORT

2. maintains its precise molecular structure and freely moves throughout the plasma in its normal gaseous state.
3. dissolved O_2
4. a. 0.15
   b. 0.15 vol%
5. the amount of O_2 in mL that is in 100 mL of blood.
6. 280
7. A
8. four

9. $Hb + O_2 \leftrightharpoons Hb_{O_2}$

10. 50, 25
11. oxyhemoglobin
12. reduced hemoglobin, deoxyhemoglobin
13. directly
14. two identical α chains, each with 141 amino acids, and two identical β chains, each with 146 amino acids ($\alpha_2\beta_2$).
15. two α, two γ
16. methemoglobin
17. a. 14–16
    b. 12–15
    c. 14–20
18. 33
19. 1.34
20. a. thebesian venous drainage into the left atrium
    b. bronchial venous drainage into the pulmonary veins
    c. alveoli that are underventilated in proportion to pulmonary blood flow
21. **Case A**
    a. 0.165
    b. 14.807
    c. 14.972
    d. 149.72
    e. 898.32
    Case B
    a. 0.15
    b. 19.296
    c. 19.446
    d. 194.46

e. 680.61
f. 12.135
g. 24.57

OXYGEN DISSOCIATION CURVE

1. percentage, pressure
2. a. the hemoglobin has an excellent safety zone for the loading of oxygen in the lungs
   b. the diffusion of oxygen during the transit time hemoglobin is in the alveolar-capillary system is enhanced
   c. increasing the P_{O_2} beyond 100 mm Hg adds very little additional oxygen to the blood
3. a. P_{O_2} reductions below 60 mm Hg indicate a rapid decrease in the amount of oxygen bound to hemoglobin
   b. a large amount of oxygen is released from the hemoglobin for only a small decrease in P_{O_2}
4. a. 85 percent
   b. 17 vol%
5. the partial pressure at which the hemoglobin is 50% saturated with oxygen.
6. 27
7. a
8. b
9. a. increased pH
      decreased P_{CO_2}
      decreased temperature
      decreased DPG
      Hb F
      CO_{Hb}
   b. decreased pH
      increased P_{CO_2}
      increased temperature
      increased DPG
10. b
11. a
12. a
13. b

OXYGEN TRANSPORT CALCULATIONS

1. a. total oxygen delivery
   b. arterial-venous oxygen content difference
   c. oxygen consumption
   d. oxygen extraction ratio
   e. mixed venous oxygen saturation
   f. pulmonary shunting
2. a. body's ability to oxygenate blood
   b. hemoglobin concentration
   c. cardiac output
3. $D_{O_2} = \dot{Q}_T \times (Ca_{O_2} \times 10)$

4. 420 mL O_2/min
5. a. decline in blood oxygenation
   b. decline in hemoglobin concentration
   c. decline in cardiac output
6. between the Ca_{O_2} and the $C\bar{v}_{O_2}$.
7. $C(a - \bar{v})_{O_2} = Ca_{O_2} - C\bar{v}_{O_2}$
8. 4 vol%
9. a. decreased cardiac output
   b. periods of increased oxygen consumption
      1. exercise
      2. seizures
      3. shivering
      4. hyperthermia
10. a. increased cardiac output
    b. skeletal muscle relaxation
    c. peripheral shunting
    d. certain poisons (cyanide)
    e. hypothermia
11. oxygen consumption, oxygen uptake
12. $\dot{V}_{O_2} = \dot{Q}_T[C(a - \bar{v})_{O_2} \times 10]$
13. 600 mL O_2/min
14. a. exercise
    b. seizures
    c. shivering
    d. hyperthermia
15. a. skeletal muscle relaxation
    b. peripheral shunting
    c. certain poisons (cyanide)
    d. hypothermia
16. body surface area (BSA)
17. 125, 165
18. extracted by the peripheral tissues divided by the amount of oxygen delivered to the peripheral cells.
19. a. oxygen coefficient ratio
    b. oxygen utilization ratio
20. $O_2ER = \dfrac{Ca_{O_2} - C\bar{v}_{O_2}}{CaO_2}$
21. 25
22. a. 50
    b. 425, 425
23. a. decreased cardiac output
    b. period of increased oxygen consumption
       1. exercise
       2. seizures
       3. shivering
       4. hyperthermia
    c. anemia
    d. decreased arterial oxygenation
24. a. increased cardiac output
    b. skeletal muscle relaxation

    c. peripheral shunting

    d. certain poisons (cyanide)

    e. hypothermia

    f. increased hemoglobin concentration

    g. increased arterial oxygenation

25. 75

26. 65

27. a. decreased cardiac output

    b. periods of increased oxygen consumption

       1. exercises

       2. seizures

       3. shivering

       4. hyperthermia

28. a

29. a. increased cardiac output

    b. skeletal muscle relaxation

    c. peripheral shunting

    d. certain poisons (cyanide)

    e. hypothermia

30. b

PULMONARY SHUNTING

1. that portion of the cardiac output that moves from the right side to the left side of the heart without being exposed to alveolar oxygen ($P_{A_{O_2}}$).
2. a. anatomic shunts
   b. capillary shunts
3. blood flows from the right side of the heart to the left side without coming in contact with an alveolus for gas exchange.
4. 3 percent
5. a. congenital heart disease
   b. intrapulmonary fistula
   c. vascular lung tumors
6. a. alveolar collapse or atelectasis
   b. alveolar fluid accumulation
   c. alveolar consolidation
7. true, absolute shunt
8. Absolute shunting is *refractory* to oxygen therapy; that is, the reduced arterial oxygen level produced by this form of pulmonary shunting cannot be treated simply by increasing the concentration of inspired oxygen, because (1) the alveoli are unable to accommodate any form of ventilation, and (2) the blood that bypasses functional alveoli cannot carry more oxygen once it has become fully saturated—except for a very small amount that dissolves in the plasma ($P_{O_2} \times 0.003 =$ dissolved O_2).
9. pulmonary capillary perfusion is in excess of alveolar ventilation.
10. a. hypoventilation
    b. ventilation/perfusion mismatches
    c. alveolar-capillary diffusion defects
11. the mixing of shunted, non-reoxygenated blood with reoxygenated blood distal to the alveoli

12. $\dfrac{\dot{Q}_S}{\dot{Q}_T} = \dfrac{Cc_{O_2} - Ca_{O_2}}{Cc_{O_2} - C\bar{v}_{O_2}}$

13. a. 268.1 mm Hg
    b. 14.204 vol% $_{O_2}$
    c. 12.389 vol% $_{O_2}$
    d. 8.139 vol% $_{O_2}$
    e. 0.29

14. a. reflects normal lung status
    b. reflects an intrapulmonary abnormality
    c. reflects significant intrapulmonary disease, and may be life threatening in patients with limited cardiovascular or central nervous system function
    d. reflects a potentially life-threatening situation—aggressive cardiopulmonary support is generally required

15. a. questionable perfusion status
    b. decreased myocardial reserve
    c. unstable oxygen consumption demand

HYPOXEMIA VERSUS HYPOXIA

1. to an abnormally low arterial oxygen tension (Pa_{O_2}) and is frequently associated with hypoxia, which is an inadequate level of tissue oxygenation.

2. a. 60–80 mm Hg
   b. 40–60 mm Hg
   c. <40 mm Hg

3. low or inadequate oxygen for cellular metabolism.

4. a. low alveolar oxygen tension
   b. diffusion effects
   c. ventilation-perfusion mismatches
   d. pulmonary shunting

5. the oxygen tension in the arterial blood is normal but the oxygen-carrying capacity of the blood is inadequate.

6. a. a low amount of hemoglobin in the blood
   b. a deficiency in the ability of hemoglobin to carry oxygen

7. the arterial blood that reaches the tissue cells may have a normal oxygen tension and content, but the amount of blood—and, therefore, the amount of oxygen—is not adequate to meet tissue needs.

8. a. slow or stagnant peripheral blood flow
   b. arterial-venous shunting

9. any condition that impairs the ability of tissue cells to utilize oxygen.

10. the term used to describe the gray or purplish discoloration seen on the mucous membranes, fingertips, and toes

11. an increased level of red blood cells

CHAPTER SEVEN

CARBON DIOXIDE TRANSPORT AND ACID-BASE BALANCE

CARBON DIOXIDE TRANSPORT

1. a. carbamino compound
   b. bicarbonate
   c. dissolved CO_2
2. a. dissolved CO_2
   b. carbamino-Hb
   c. bicarbonate
3. bicarbonate
4. 63

CARBON DIOXIDE DISSOCIATION CURVE

1. linear
2. 40, 50
3. Haldane effect

ACID-BASE BALANCE AND REGULATION

1. 7.35, 7.45
2. 7.30, 7.40
3. alkalosis, alkalemia
4. acidosis, acidemia
5. a. the breakdown of phosphorous-containing proteins (phosphoric acid)
   b. the anaerobic metabolism of glucose (lactic acid)
   c. the metabolism of body fats (fatty and ketone acids)
   d. the transport of CO_2 in the blood as HCO_3^- liberates H^+ ions.
6. a. the chemical buffer system
   b. the respiratory system
   c. the renal system
7. first line of defense
8. H^+ ions, HCO_3^- ions, alkalosis
9. 1, 3, depth, rate

10. most effective acid-base balance monitor and regulator
11. day or more
12. HCO3⁻, H⁺, increase
13. retains H⁺, excretes basic substances (primarily HCO_3^-), decrease

The Basic Principles of Acid-Base Reactions and pH

Acids and Bases

1. acids and bases are electrolytes.
   a. ionize and dissociate in water
   b. conduct an electrical current

Acids

1. releases hydrogen ions [H⁺]
2. proton donors
3. free hydrogen ions
4. $HCl \rightarrow$ H⁺   Cl⁻
            proton   anion

Strong and Weak Acids

1. free hydrogen ions, hydrogen ions still combined with anions
2. completely, they liberate all the H⁺, irreversibly
3. 100 H⁺, 100 Cl⁻.
4. not dissociate completely
5. carbonic acid (H_2CO_3), acetic acid (HAc).
6. $100 \ HC_2H_3O_2 \rightarrow 90 \ HC_2H_3O_2 + 10 \ H^+ + 10 \ C_2H_3O_2^-$

Bases

1. proton acceptors
2. takes up hydrogen ions [H⁺]
3. hydroxide ions (OH⁻) and cations
4. $NaOH \rightarrow$ Na⁺ +   OH⁻
                cation   hydroxyl ion
   and then $OH^- + H^+ \rightarrow H_2O$
                                      water
5. bicarbonate ion (HCO_3^-)
6. ammonia (NH_3), ammonia (NH_3)

Strong and Weak Bases

1. proton acceptors
2. H^+
3. dissociate incompletely, reversibly, slower to accept protons
4. as a weak base.

pH: Acid-Base Concentration

1. hydrogen ions
2. hydroxide ions
3. pH units
4. 0 to 14, logarithmic
5. tenfold
6. the negative logarithm, to the base 10, of the hydrogen ion concentration $[H^+]$ in moles per liter, or $-\log H^+$

$$pH = -\log_{10} [H^+]$$

7. hydrogen ions precisely equals the number of hydroxide ions (OH^-), acidic, basic.
8. 7, 10^{-7} mol/L (0.0000001 mol/L) of hydrogen
9. acidic, more hydrogen ions than hydroxide
10. 10 times more hydrogen, 7
11. alkaline, hydroxide ions outnumber the hydrogen
12. 10 times more hydroxide, 7
13. falls

The Chemical Buffer Systems and Acid-Base Balance

1. first line of defense
2. buffer action.
3. releasing hydrogen ions (acting as acids) when the pH increases, binding hydrogen ions (acting as bases) when the pH decreases.
4. carbonic acid-bicarbonate buffer system, the phosphate buffer system, and the protein buffer system.

Carbonic Acid-Bicarbonate Buffer System and Acid-Base Balance

1.
	Response to an increase in pH		
H_2CO_3	$\rightleftharpoons$	HCO_3^-	$+$ H^+
H^+ donor	Response to a decrease in pH	H^+ acceptor	proton
(weak acid)		(weak proton)	

2. a. strong bases to a weak base (bicarbonate ion)
   b. strong acids to a weak acid (carbonic acid)

The Henderson-Hasselbalch Equation

1. $pH = pK + \log \dfrac{[HCO_3^-]}{[H_2CO_3]}$
2. the dissociation constant of the acid portion of the buffer combination
3. $6:1$
4. $20:1$
5. b
6. c

Phosphate Buffer System and Acid-Base Balance

1. sodium salts of dihydrogen phosphate ($H_2PO_4^-$), monohydrogen phosphate (HPO_4^{2-})
2. acid
3. base
4. one-sixth

Protein Buffer System and Acid-Base Balance

1. proteins in the plasma, cells
2. 75 percent
3. polymers
4. organic acid (carboxyl) groups (—COOH), liberate H^+, rising pH
5. accept H^+
6. amphoteric molecules
7. intracellular buffer
8. H_2CO_3, H^+, HCO_3^-, reduced hemoglobin
9. True
10. False

The Respiratory System and Acid-Base Balance

1. two
2. $CO_2 + H_2O \leftrightarrows H_2CO_3 \leftrightarrows H^+ + HCO_3^-$
3. True
4. increasing
5. decreasing
6. False
7. True

The Renal System and Acid-Base Balance

1. phosphoric acids, uric acids, lactic acids, ketone acids.
2. alkaline substances, restore chemical buffers
3. retains HCO_3^-, H^+, increase
4. retains H^+, basic, decrease

THE ROLE OF THE P_{CO_2}/HCO_3^-/pH RELATIONSHIP IN ACID-BASE BALANCE

Acid-Base Balance Disturbances

1. a. increase
   b. increase
   c. increase
   d. decrease
   e. decrease
2. a. decrease
   b. decrease
   c. decrease
   d. increase
   e. increase

Respiratory Acid-Base Disturbances

Acute Ventilatory Failure (Respiratory Acidosis)

1. 7.22, 27 mEq/L
2. a. chronic obstructive pulmonary disorders
   b. drug overdose
   c. general anesthesia
   d. head trauma
   e. neurologic disorders

Renal Compensation

1. b
2. 38 mEq/L or greater

Acute Alveolar Hyperventilation (Respiratory Alkalosis)

1. 7.60, 20 mEq/L
2. a. hypoxia
   b. pain, anxiety, fever
   c. brain inflammation
   d. stimulant drugs

Renal Compensation

1. e
2. 16 mEq/L or less

Metabolic Acid-Base Imbalances

Metabolic Acidosis

1. 13 mEq/L
2. a. lactic acidosis
   b. ketoacidosis
   c. salicylate intoxication
   d. renal failure
   e. uncontrolled diarrhea

Anion Gap

1. a. 140 mEq/L
   b. 105 mEq/L
   c. 24 mEq/L
2. 13 mEq/L
3. 14 mEq/L
4. fixed acids (e.g., lactic acid, ketoacids, or salicylate intoxication)
5. hyperchloremic metabolic acidosis

Metabolic Acidosis with Respiratory Compensation

1. c
2. 15 mm Hg or less
3. e

Metabolic Alkalosis

1. 39 mEq/L
2. a. hypokalemia
   b. hypochloremia
   c. gastric suction or vomiting
   d. excessive administration of corticosteroids
   e. excessive administration of sodium bicarbonate
   f. diuretic therapy
   g. hypovolemia

Metabolic Alkalosis with Respiratory Compensation

1. g
2. 75 mm Hg or less
3. i

CHAPTER EIGHT

VENTILATION-PERFUSION RELATIONSHIPS

VENTILATION-PERFUSION RATIO

1. 4
2. 5
3. 4, 5, 0.8
4. higher
5. lower
6. decreases
7. a. the amount of oxygen ventilated into the alveoli
   b. the amount of oxygen removed by capillary blood flow
8. a. the amount of carbon dioxide that diffuses into the alveoli from the capillary blood
   b. the amount of carbon dioxide removed from the alveoli by means of ventilation
9. it washes out of the alveoli faster than it is replaced by the venous blood.
10. it does not diffuse into the blood as fast as it enters the alveolus. The $P_{A_{O_2}}$ also increases because of the reduced $P_{A_{CO_2}}$.
11. a
12. oxygen moves out of the alveolus and into the pulmonary capillary blood faster than it is replenished by ventilation.
13. it moves out of the capillary blood and into the alveolus faster than it is washed out of the alveolus.
14. c
15. decreases
16. increases
17. decreases
18. gas exchange between the systemic capillaries and the tissue cells.
19. 250
20. 200
21. ratio between the volume of oxygen consumed and the volume of carbon dioxide produced.

22. $RQ = \dfrac{\dot{V}_{CO_2}}{\dot{V}_{O_2}}$

23. gas exchange between the pulmonary capillaries and the alveoli.
24. quantity of oxygen and carbon dioxide exchanged during a period of 1 minute.
25. a. pulmonary emboli
    b. partial or complete obstruction in the pulmonary artery or arterioles
    c. extrinsic pressure on the pulmonary vessels
    d. destruction of the pulmonary vessels
    e. decreased cardiac output
26. a. obstructive lung disorder
    b. restrictive lung disorders
    c. hypoventilation from any cause

CHAPTER NINE

CONTROL OF VENTILATION

THE RESPIRATORY COMPONENTS OF THE MEDULLA OBLONGATA

1. a. dorsal respiratory group
   b. ventral respiratory group
2. a
3. c
4. b

THE INFLUENCE OF THE PONTINE RESPIRATORY CENTERS ON THE RESPIRATORY COMPONENTS OF THE MEDULLA OBLONGATA

1. the lower pons
2. b
3. b

MONITORING SYSTEMS THAT INFLUENCE THE RESPIRATORY COMPONENTS OF THE MEDULLA OBLONGATA

1. hydrogen ions [H^+]
2. bilaterally and ventrally in the substance of the medulla
3. CO_2, H^+, HCO_3^-
4. $CO_2 + H_2O \leftrightarrows H_2CO_3 \leftrightarrows H^+ + HCO_3^-$
5. The central chemoreceptors transmit signals to the respiratory component in the medulla, which, in turn, increases alveolar ventilation.
6. indirect, pH level of the CSF
7. special oxygen-sensitive cells that react to reductions of oxygen levels in the arterial blood.
8. high in the neck at the bifurcation of the internal and external carotid arteries and on the aortic arch
9. glossopharyngeal (ninth); vagus (tenth)

10. a
11. 60 mm Hg
12. 30 mm Hg
13. A chronically high CO_2 concentration in the CSF inactivates the H^+ sensitivity of the central chemoreceptors. HCO_3^- moves into the CSF via the active transport mechanism and combines with H^+, thus returning the pH to normal.
14. a
15. a. chronic anemia
    b. carbon monoxide poisoning
    c. methemoglobinemia
16. a. decreased pH (increased H^+ level)
    b. hypoperfusion
    c. increased temperature
    d. nicotine
    e. the direct effect of Pa_{CO_2}
17. a. peripheral vasoconstriction
    b. increased pulmonary vascular resistance
    c. systemic arterial hypertension
    d. tachycardia
    e. increase in left ventricular performance

REFLEXES THAT INFLUENCE VENTILATION

1. lung overinflation
2. inspiration to cease.
3. lung compression or deflation
4. an increased rate of breathing
5. lung exposure to noxious gases or accumulated mucus
6. in the trachea, bronchi, and bronchioles
7. the ventilatory rate to increase.
8. small conducting airways, blood vessels, and interstitial tissues between the pulmonary capillaries and alveolar walls
9. juxtapulmonary-capillary receptors, or J-receptors
10. alveolar inflammation, pulmonary capillary congestion and edema, humoral agents (e.g., serotonin and bradykinin), lung deflation, and emboli
11. rapid, shallow breathing pattern
12. muscles, tendons, joints, and pain receptors in muscles and skin
13. medulla, increased number of inspiratory signals
14. increased respiratory rate during exercise
15. greater
16. increase
17. increase
18. a decreased heart and ventilatory rate.
19. an increased heart and ventilatory rate.

CHAPTER TEN

FETAL DEVELOPMENT AND THE CARDIOPULMONARY SYSTEM

FETAL LUNG DEVELOPMENT

1. a. embryonic
   b. pseudoglandular
   c. canalicular
   d. terminal sac
2. 24th
3. 20
4. 28th

PLACENTA

1. cotyledons
2. (Fig. 10-3, pg. 364)
3. umbilical arteries
4. 20, 55
5. The decreased maternal P_{CO_2} is caused by the alveolar hyperventilation that develops as the growing infant restricts the mother's diaphragmatic excursion.
6. a. maternal-fetal P_{O_2} gradient
   b. higher hemoglobin concentration in the fetal blood
   c. greater affinity of fetal hemoglobin for oxygen
7. 30, 40
8. umbilical vein
9. a. The placenta itself is an actively metabolizing organ.
   b. The permeability of the placenta varies from region to region with respect to respiratory gases.
   c. There are fetal and maternal vascular shunts.

FETAL CIRCULATION

1. ductus venosus
2. foramen ovale
3. left ventricle, heart, brain
4. ductus arteriosus, aorta
5. 15, pulmonary veins
6. 20
7. e
   c
   a
   b
   d
8. a. The placenta is passed by the mother.
   b. The umbilical arteries atrophy and become the lateral umbilical ligaments.
   c. The umbilical vein becomes the round ligament (ligamentum teres) of the liver.
   d. The ductus venosus becomes the ligamentum venosum, which is a fibrous cord in the liver.
   e. The flap on the foramen ovale usually closes and becomes a depression in the interatrial septum called the fossa ovalis.
   f. The ductus arteriosus atrophies and becomes the ligamentum arteriosum.
9. a. About one-third of the fluid is squeezed out of the lungs as the infant passes through the birth canal.
   b. About one-third of the fluid is absorbed by the pulmonary capillaries.
   c. About one-third of the fluid is removed by the lymphatic system.
10. 24
11. 12

BIRTH

1. a. thermal
   b. tactile
   c. visual
2. -40
3. 40
4. 0.005 L/cm H_2O
5. 30 cm H_2O/L/sec
6. a. The sudden increase in the alveolar P_{O_2}, which offsets the hypoxic vasoconstriction.
   b. The removal of fluid from the lungs, reducing the external pressure on the pulmonary vessels.
   c. The mechanical increase in lung volume, which widens the caliber of the extra-alveolar vessels.
7. As the pulmonary vascular resistance decreases, a greater amount of blood flows through the lungs, and, therefore, more blood returns to the left atrium. This causes the pressure in the left atrium to increase and the flap of the foramen ovale to close.
8. 45, 50
9. When the ductus arteriosus remains open (permitting blood to pass through it) and the pulmonary vascular resistance is elevated, persistent pulmonary hypertension of the neonate is said to exist.
10. persistent fetal circulation

11. a. bradykinin
    b. serotonin
    c. prostaglandin inhibitors

CONTROL OF VENTILATION IN THE NEWBORN

1. peripheral, central
2. decrease
3. respiratory slowing or apnea
4. marked hyperventilation
5. a deep inspiration that is elicited by lung inflation

CHAPTER ELEVEN

AGING AND THE CARDIOPULMONARY SYSTEM

THE EFFECTS OF AGING ON THE RESPIRATORY SYSTEM

1. 20
2. 20, 25
3. decreases, increases
4. a. increases
   b. decreases
   c. decreases
   d. remains the same
   e. increases
   f. increases
   g. decreases
5. a. decreases
   b. decreases
   c. decreases
   d. decreases
   e. decreases
   f. decreases
   g. decreases
6. a. decreases
   b. increases
   c. increases
   d. decreases
   e. remains the same
   f. remains the same
   g. remains the same
   h. decreases
   i. decreases

ARTERIAL BLOOD GASES

1. b
2. a. decreases
   b. decreases
3. b

THE EFFECTS OF AGING ON THE CARDIOVASCULAR SYSTEM

1. b
2. b
3. b
4. 150 beats/min.
5. a. decreases
   b. decreases
   c. increases
   d. increases
   e. increases
   f. decreases

CHAPTER TWELVE

ELECTROPHYSIOLOGY OF THE HEART

ELECTROPHYSIOLOGY OF THE HEART

1. action potentials
2. polarized or resting state
3. resting membrane potential (RMP)
4. potassium (K^+), sodium (Na^+), and calcium (Ca^{2+})
5. greatest
6. K^+ cation, Na^+ cation
7. -90 mV
8. action potential

THE FIVE PHASES OF THE ACTION POTENTIAL

1. Na^+, Na^+ channels; positively charged
2. $+30$ mV; up-stroke.
3. K^+, K^+, out
4. downward
5. inward, Ca^{2+}, outward, K^+
6. prolonged
7. inward, Ca^{2+}, outward, K^+
8. Na^+, K^+, Na^+, K^+

PROPERTIES OF THE CARDIAC MUSCLE

1. contractile muscle fibers, autorhythmic cells.
2. contractile fiber cells
3. sinoatrial node
4. into, 4
5. more, less
6. transmit, cell to cell
7. shorten and contract

Refractory Periods

1. cannot respond to a stimulus
2. 0, 1, 2, and about half of phase 3
3. strong
4. 3
5. resting or polarized state
6. 4

The Conductive System

1. See Figure 12-4, pg. 402

Autonomic Nervous System

1. heart rate, AV conduction, cardiac contractility, and excitability
2. heart rate, AV conduction, contractility, and excitability

CHAPTER THIRTEEN

THE STANDARD 12-ECG SYSTEM

THE STANDARD 12-ECG SYSTEM

1. four, six
2. See Table 13-1 in textbook (ref. pg. 408)
3. a. views the electrical activity of the heart from a different angle
   b. has a positive and negative component
   c. monitors specific portions of the heart from the point of view of the positive electrode in that lead

Standard Limb Leads

1. bipolar leads, positive, negative
2. axis
3. Einthoven's triangle
4. positive deflections
5. equiphasic, straight
6. negative
7. base, apex, right, left
8. positive, zero, center; center, negative; electrode, center
9. 50 percent; augmentation; voltage; positive electrode is placed
10. frontal plane, base to the apex of the heart, right, left
11. left lateral leads; inferior leads

Precordial (Chest) Leads

1. horizontal plane; right ventricle; ventricle septum, left ventricle
2. anterior leads; lateral leads

Modified Chest Lead

1. V1; left arm or left shoulder area

NORMAL ECG CONFIGURATIONS AND THEIR EXPECTED MEASUREMENTS (LEAD II)

The ECG Paper

1. 0.04; five, 0.20
2. 5, 300
3. amplitude, 0.1, 1
4. 10
5. 15, 3
6. baseline; it changes into another wave form
7. complex
8. segment
9. interval
10. positive; negative

The P Wave

1. P wave
2. symmetric, upright
3. AV node
4. flat, isoelectic
5. 0.08, 0.11, 2 to 2½
6. 0.2, 0.3, 2 to 3
7. atrial abnormalities
8. ventricles are depolarizing

The PR Interval

1. P wave, QRS complex
2. 0.12, 0.20, 3, 5
3. bundle of His, ventricular branches, Purkinje fiber system

The QRS Complex

1. ventricular depolarization
2. Q wave, R wave, S wave
3. Q wave
4. R wave
5. S
6. 0.10, 2½
7. longer, 0.10
8. premature ventricular contractions (PVCs), increased amplitude, T waves of opposite polarity

The ST Segment

1. ventricular depolarization, repolarization
2. QRS complex (called the J point), T wave
3. 0.12
4. ischemia

The T Wave

1. ventricular repolarization, rest, and recovery
2. 0.5
3. 0.20
4. refractory period
5. relative refractory
6. acid-base imbalances, hyperventilation, hyperkalemia, ischemia, and the presence of various drugs

The U Wave

1. T wave, T wave
2. flat and not seen

The QT Interval

1. QRS complex, T wave
2. total ventricular activity—that is, ventricular depolarization (QRS) and repolarization (ST segment and the T wave)
3. 0.38
4. 40 percent
5. indirectly

CHAPTER FOURTEEN

ECG INTERPRETATION

HOW TO ANALYZE THE WAVEFORMS

Step One: Does the General Appearance of the ECG Tracing Appear Normal or Abnormal?

1. Closely scan the ECG tracing and identify each of the wave components. Note any specific wave abnormalities. Are there any abnormalities—in terms of appearance or duration—in the P waves, QRS complexes, ST segments, or T waves? Do the complexes appear consistent from one beat to the next? Does the rate appear too slow or too fast? Does the rhythm appear regular or irregular? Are there any extra beats or pauses? It is often helpful to circle any possible abnormalities during Step 1. This initial process helps to pinpoint problem areas that can be inspected more carefully during the steps discussed next.

Step Two: Does the Ventricular Activity (QRS Complexes) Appear Normal or Abnormal?

Rate

1. large, QRS complexes, 300, large
2. See Table 14-2 (ref. pg. 427)
3. vertical 3-second marks
4. 6-second interval (two 3-second marks), 10

Rhythm

1. shortest; longest
2. 0.12

Shape

1. 0.10, 2½ small squares or less
2. supraventricular origin
3. 0.10, distorted

Step Three: Does the Atrial Activity Appear Normal or Abnormal?

1. QRS complexes
2. the same
3. QRS rhythm, PP intervals
4. P waves that are not of expected polarity, atrial flutter, fibrillation, or P prime (P') waves (i.e., waves initiated outside SA node)

Step Four: Does the Atrioventricular Relationship Appear to Be Normal?

1. all the atrial impulses
2. a. Is each P wave followed by a QRS complex?
   b. Is each QRS complex preceded by a single P wave?
3. 0.20

Step Five: What Is the ECG Interpretation?

1. P wave	The P waves are positive (upright) and uniform. A QRS complex follows every P wave.
PR interval:	The duration of the PR interval is between 0.12 and 0.20 second and is constant from beat to beat.
QRS complex	The duration of the QRS complex is 0.10 second or less. A P wave precedes every QRS complex.
QRS rate:	Between 60 and 100 beats per minute.
QRS rhythm:	Regular

COMMON CARDIAC DYSRHYTHMIAS

The Sinus Mechanisms

Sinus Bradycardia

1. slow
2. 60
3.

P wave:	The P waves are positive and uniform. Each P wave is followed by a QRS complex.
PR interval:	The PR interval has a normal duration between 0.12 and 0.20 second and is constant from beat to beat.
QRS complex:	The QRS complex duration is 0.10 second or less. A P wave precedes every QRS complex.
QRS rate:	Less than 60 beats per minute.
QRS rhythm:	Regular

4. a weakened or damaged sinoatrial (SA) node, severe or chronic hypoxemia, increased intracranial pressure, obstructive sleep apnea, and certain drugs (most notably the beta-blockers)
5. decreased, lowered
6. decreased, hypoxia

Sinus Tachycardia

1. fast
2. 100, 160
3.

P wave:	The P waves are positive and uniform. Each P wave is followed by a QRS complex.
PR interval:	The PR interval has a normal duration between 0.12 and 0.20 second and is constant from beat to beat.
QRS complex:	The QRS complex duration is 0.10 second or less. A P wave precedes every QRS complex.
QRS rate:	Between 100 and 160 beats per minute.
QRS rhythm:	Regular

4. exercise, emotions, fever, pain, fear, anger, and anxiety
5. hypoxemia, hypovolemia, severe anemia, hyperthermia, massive hemorrhage, hyperthyroidism, and any condition that leads to an increased sympathetic stimulation
6. congestive heart failure, cardiogenic shock, myocardial ischemia, heart valve disorders, pulmonary embolism, hypertension, and infarction

Sinus Arrhythmia

1. 10
2. normal
3.

P wave:	The P waves are positive and uniform. Each P wave is followed by a QRS complex.
PR interval:	The PR interval has a normal duration between 0.12 and 0.20 second and is constant from beat to beat.
QRS complex:	The QRS complex duration is 0.10 second or less. A P wave precedes every QRS complex.
QRS rate:	Varies by more than 10 percent.
QRS rhythm:	Irregular

4. children, young adults.

Sinus (SA) Block

1. sinus exit block, blocked.
2. at the precise time it would normally appear if the sinus block had not occurred
3.

P wave:	The P waves are positive and uniform. However, there is an entire P-QRS-T complex missing.
PR interval:	The PR interval has a normal duration between 0.12 and 0.20 second and is constant from beat to beat, except for the pause when an entire cycle is missing. The PR interval may be slightly shorter after the pause.

QRS complex:	Except for the missing cycle, the QRS complex duration is 0.10 second or less, and a P wave precedes every QRS complex.
QRS rate:	The rate may vary according to the number and position of missing P-QRS-T cycles.
QRS rhythm:	The rhythm may be regular or irregular according to the number and position of missing P-QRS-T cycles.

Sinus Arrest

1. sudden failure of the SA node to initiate an impulse (i.e., no P-wave)
2.

P wave:	No P wave.
PR interval:	The PR interval has a normal duration between 0.12 and 0.20 second and is constant from beat to beat.
QRS complex:	The QRS complex duration is 0.10 second or less. After a sinus arrest, however, the QRS duration may be greater than 0.10 second when the escape rhythm is initiated by the AV node.
QRS rate:	Normal sinus rhythm during nonsinus arrest periods.
QRS rhythm:	The QRS complexes before and after the sinus arrest are regular. The escape rate may be regular or irregular.

The Atrial Mechanisms

Premature Atrial Complex

1. abnormal electrical activity in the atria cause the atria to depolarize before the SA node fires
2. ectopic foci
3. P prime (P′)
4.

P wave:	The P′ wave will appear different from a normal SA node-induced P wave. The P′ may be hidden, or partially hidden, in the preceding T wave. P′ waves hidden in the T wave often distort or increase the amplitude of the T wave. A PAC may not successfully move into the ventricles if the AV node or bundle branches are in their complete refractory period. This is called a blocked or nonconducted PAC.
PR interval:	The P′R interval may be normal or prolonged, depending on the timing of the PAC. Most often, however, the P′R interval is different from the normal SA node rhythm.
QRS complex:	The QRS complex duration is 0.10 second or less, and a normal P wave precedes every QRS complex.
QRS rate:	Varies
QRS rhythm:	Irregular

5. hypoxemia impending heart failure, right coronary artery disease, digitalis excess, pericarditis, ingestion of stimulants or caffeine, and recreational drug abuse
6. a. patients with chronic obstructive pulmonary lung disease
   b. females during the third trimester of pregnancy

Atrial Bigeminy

1. every other beat is an ectopic atrial beat—a PAC
2. congestive heart failure

Atrial Tachycardia

1. 130, 250
2. paroxysmal atrial tachycardia
3. P' wave: Starts abruptly, at rates of 130 to 250 beats per minute. The P' wave may or may not be seen. Visible P' waves differ in configuration from the normal sinus P wave. At more rapid rates, the P' is hidden in the preceding T wave and cannot be seen as a separate entity.
   P'R interval: The P'R interval has a normal duration between 0.12 and 0.20 second and is constant from beat to beat. The P'R interval is difficult to measure at rapid rates.
   QRS complex: The QRS complex duration is 0.10 second or less. A P wave usually precedes every QRS complex, although a 2:1 AV conduction ratio is often seen. The QRS complexes during atrial tachycardia may be normal or abnormal, depending on the degree of ventricular refractoriness and AV conduction time.
   QRS rate: Very regular
   QRS rhythm: Atrial trachycardia begins suddenly and is very regular.
4. anxiety, caffeine, smoking, and excessive alcohol ingestion

Atrial Flutter

1. two or more regular "sawtooth-like" waves, called flutter or ff waves
2. 200, 300
3. ff waves: Atrial depolarization is regular. Commonly has a sawtooth-like or sharktooth-like appearance.
   P'R interval: The P'R interval of the ff waves is typically between 0.24 to 0.40 second and consistent with the QRS complex.
   QRS complex: The QRS complex duration is usually 0.10 second or less. Depending on the degree of ventricular refractoriness, the QRS may be greater than 0.10 second. When this is the case, the ff waves distort the QRS complexes and T waves.
   QRS rate: The QRS rate is a function of the degree of ventricular refractoriness and of the AV conduction time.
   QRS rhythm: Depending on AV conduction, the QRS rhythm may be regular or irregular.
4. 40, chronic obstructive pulmonary disease (e.g., emphysema or chronic bronchitis), chronic heart disease (e.g., congestive heart failure or valvular heart disease), chronic hypertension, myocardial ischemia, myocardial infarction, hypoxemia, quinidine excess, pulmonary embolus, and hepatic disease

Atrial Fibrillation

1. disorganized, and ineffective state within the atria
2. coarse fibrillation

3. 300, 600
4. fib, ff waves.
5. ff waves: Atrial depolarization is chaotic and irregular.
   PR interval: here are no PR intervals.
   QRS complex: The QRS complex duration is usually 0.10 second or less. The ff waves often distort the QRS complexes and T waves.
   QRS rate: The QRS rate is a function of the degree of ventricular refractoriness and conduction time.
   QRS rhythm: Depending on AV conduction, the QRS rhythm may be regular or irregular.
6. chronic obstructive pulmonary disease, valvular heart disease, congestive heart failure, ischemic heart disease, and hypertensive heart disorders
7. emotional stress, excessive alcohol consumption, and excessive straining and vomiting

The Ventricular Mechanisms

Premature Ventricular Complex (PVC)

1. abnormal electrical activity arising within the ventricles
2. P wave: There is no P wave before a PVC. The P waves of the dominant rhythm are normal.
   PR interval: There is no PR interval before a PVC. The PR intervals of the dominant rhythm are normal.
   QRS complex: The QRS complex is wide (long duration), bizarre, and unlike the normal QRS complex. The QRS of the PVC usually has an increased amplitude with a T wave of opposite polarity. The QRS-T may also present with diminished amplitude and narrow duration.
   QRS rate: The QRS rate is that of the underlying rhythm
   QRS rhythm: The rhythm is that of the underlying rhythm, and PVCs disturb the regularity.
3. uniform PVCs, multiform PVCs, paried PVCs, bigeminal PVCs, trigeminal PVCs.
4. from one focus; appearance, size and amplitude
5. more than one focus; shapes and amplitudes
6. two closely coupled PVCs in a row
7. every other beat—that is, a normal sinus beat, PVC, sinus beat, PVC, and so on
8. when every third beat is a PVC
9. intrinsic myocardial disease, electrolyte disturbances, hypoxemia, acidemia, hypokalemia, hypertension, hypovolemia, stress, and congestive heart failure
10. digitalis, isoproterenol, dopamine, epinephrine, and caffeine. PVCs may also be a sign of theophylline or alpha-or beta-agonist toxicity.

Ventricular Tachycardia

1. ventricular tachycardia
2. 100, 170
3. paroxysmal, intermittent

4. sustained ventricular tachycardia, V-tach
5. decreased
6. P wave   The P wave usually cannot be identified during ventricular tachycardia.
   PR interval: The PR interval cannot be measured.
   QRS complex: The QRS duration is usually greater than 0.12 second and bizarre in appear-
                   ance. The T wave usually cannot be identified.
   QRS rate: Between 100 and 170 beats per minute. Three or more consecutive PVCs con-
                   stitute ventricular tachycardia.
   QRS rhythm: Regular or slightly irregular.

Ventricular Flutter

1. QRS complexes
2. 250, 350
3. P wave: The P wave is usually not distinguishable.
   PR interval: The PR interval is not measurable.
   QRS complex: The QRS duration is usually greater than 0.12 second and bizarre in appear-
                   ance. The T wave is usually not separated from the QRS complex.
   QRS rate: Between 250 and 350 beats per minute.
   QRS rhythm: Regular or slightly irregular.

Ventricular Fibrillation

1. multiple and chaotic electrical activities of the ventricles
2. terminal
3. P wave: The P waves cannot be identified.
   PR interval: The PR interval is not measurable.
   QRS complex: The QRS complex cannot be identified.
   QRS rate: A rate cannot be calculated.
   QRS rhythm: The rhythm is chaotic because of multiple, disorganized ventricular contrac-
                   tions.

Asystole (Cardiac Standstill)

1. complete absence of electrical and mechanical activity
2. a flat line, severe damage to the heart's electrical conduction system

AV Conduction Defects

Sinus Rhythm with First-Degree AV Block

1. increases
2. first-degree AV block

3. P wave:

> The P waves are positive and uniform. Each P wave is followed by a QRS complex.

   PR interval:

> The PR interval is consistently greater than 0.20 second from beat to beat.

   QRS complex:

> The duration of the QRS complex is 0.10 second or less. Each QRS complex is preceded by a P wave.

   QRS rate:

> The rate is usually based upon the normal sinus rhythm and is constant between 60 and 100 per minute.

   QRS rhythm:

> The rhythm is dependent on the sinus rhythm. When a sinus arrhythmia is present, the rhythm will vary accordingly.

4. right coronary artery disease, endocarditis, myocarditis, electrolyte disturbances, and advancing age

Sinus Rhythm with Second-Degree AV Block: The Wenckebach Phenomenon

1. progressive delay in the conduction of the atrial impulse through the AV junction until, eventually, an atrial impulse is completely blocked from the ventricles
2. Progressive prolongation of the PR interval
   The complex Wenckebach cycle begins and ends with a P wave
   There is one more P wave than QRS complexes in a cycle
   Irregular or decreasing RR intervals

Complete AV Block

1. blocked
2. His bundle, 40 to 60; escape junctional pacemaker.
3. ventricular escape mechanism
4. 20 and 40
5. P wave:

> The P waves are positive and uniform. There is no relationship between the P waves and the QRS complexes. The atrial rate is faster than the ventricular escape rate.

   PR interval:

> There are no measurable PR intervals, as there is no relationship between the P waves and QRS complexes.

   QRS complex:

> The duration of the QRS complex may be normal, or greater than 0.12 second. When the pathology is above the His bundle, the QRS complex is usually normal (0.10 or less). When the pathology is below the His bundle, the duration of the QRS complexes will be greater than 0.12 second.

   QRS rate:

> The atrial rate is faster and completely independent of the ventricular rate. A junctional escape pacemaker produces a rate between 40 and 60 beats per minute. A ventricular escape pacemaker produces a rate between 20 and 40 beats per minute.

   QRS rhythm:

> Both a junctional escape pacemaker or a ventricular escape pacemaker produce a regular rhythm.

CHAPTER FIFTEEN

HEMODYNAMIC MEASUREMENTS

HEMODYNAMIC MEASUREMENTS DIRECTLY OBTAINED BY MEANS OF THE PULMONARY ARTERY CATHETER

1. the study of the forces that influence the circulation of blood.

HEMODYNAMIC VALUES COMPUTED FROM DIRECT MEASUREMENTS

2. the volume of blood ejected by the ventricles with each contraction.
3. a. preload
   b. afterload
   c. myocardial contractility

4. $SV = \dfrac{CO}{HR}$

5. 63.21 mL/beat
7. dividing the stroke volume (SV) by the body surface area (BSA).
8. 22 mL/beat/m^2
9. a. contractility of the heart
   b. overall blood volume status
   c. degree of venous return
10. dividing the cardiac output (CO) by the body's surface area (BSA).
11. 2.8 L/min/m^2
12. the amount of work required by the right ventricle to pump blood
13. contractility of the right ventricle
14. RVSWI = SVI $\times$ (PA − CVP) $\times$ 0.0136 g/mL
15. 8.16 g mm
16. the amount of work required by the left ventricle to pump blood
17. contractility of the left ventricle
18. LVSWI = SVI $\times$ (MAP − PCWP) $\times$ 0.0136 g/mL
19. 70.38 g m/m^2
20. low-
21. high-
22. the afterload of the right ventricle

23. $PVR = \dfrac{PA - PCWP \times 80}{CO}$

24. 114 dynes $\times$ sec cm^{-5}

25. the afterload of the left ventricle

26. $SVR = \dfrac{MAP - CVP \times 80}{CO}$

27. 1266 dynes $\times$ sec cm^{-5}

CHAPTER SIXTEEN

RENAL FAILURE AND ITS EFFECTS ON THE CARDIOPULMONARY SYSTEM

THE KIDNEYS

1. (ref. Fig. 16-2, pg. 476)
2. (ref. Fig. 16-3, pg. 477)
3. (ref. Fig. 16-4, pg. 479)

URINE FORMATION

1. (ref. Table 16-1, pg. 480)
2. a. proximal convoluted tubule
   b. loop of Henle
   c. distal convoluted tubule
3. proximal convoluted tubule
4. various substances are transported from the plasma of the peritubular capillaries to the fluid of the renal tubule.
5. hydrogen (H^+), potassium (K^+)

URINE CONCENTRATION AND VOLUME

1. a. countercurrent mechanism
   b. selective permeability of the collecting ducts
2. renal medulla
3. 300
4. 300, 1200
5. hypothalamus, pituitary gland
6. b
7. increases
8. a
9. decreases
10. 1.003, 1.030

REGULATION OF ELECTROLYTE CONCENTRATION

1. a. sodium
   b. potassium
   c. calcium, magnesium, and phosphate

ROLE OF THE KIDNEYS IN ACID-BASE BALANCE

1. hydrogen
2. sodium bicarbonate

BLOOD VOLUME

1. a. capillary fluid shift system
   b. the renal system

RENAL FAILURE

1. a. unilateral renal agenesis
   b. renal dysplasia
   c. polycystic disease of the kidney
2. women
3. a. calculi
   b. normal pregnancy
   c. prostatic hypertrophy
   d. infection and inflammation causing scar tissue
   e. neurologic disorders (ref. Table 16-2, pg. 487)
4. a. altered immune responses
   b. drugs and related chemicals
   c. radiation
5. Wilms' tumor
6. a. hypovolemia
   b. septicemia
   c. heart failure
   d. renal artery atherosclerosis (ref. Table 16-3, pg. 488)
7. a sharp reduction in urine output
8. a. renal ischemia
   b. injury to the glomerular membrane caused by nephrotoxic agents
   c. acute tubular necrosis
   d. intratubular obstruction
   e. acute inflammatory conditions (ref. Table 16-4, pg. 488)

9. a. ureteral obstruction
   b. bladder outlet obstruction (ref. Table 16-5, pg. 488)
10. decreases
11. increases
12. a
13. b

CARDIOPULMONARY DISORDERS CAUSED BY RENAL FAILURE

1. sodium
2. a. increases
   b. increases
   c. decreases
3. b
4. b
5. a
6. a
7. a. the production of erythropoietin is often inadequate to stimulate the production of red blood cells
   b. toxic waste accumulation suppresses the ability of bone marrow to produce red blood cells
8. because of the platelet abnormalities associated with renal failure
9. This condition develops as a result of the exposure of the pericardium to the metabolic end-products associated with renal decline

CHAPTER SEVENTEEN

SLEEP PHYSIOLOGY AND ITS RELATIONSHIP TO THE CARDIOPULMONARY SYSTEM

1. coma
2. large, small
3. polysomnogram
4. a. electroencephalogram
   b. electrooculogram
   c. electromyogram
5. a. the presence or absence of snoring
   b. nasal and oral airflow
   c. chest movement
   d. abdomen movement
   e. SaO_2
   f. electrocardiogram
6. 30 seconds

TYPES OF SLEEP

1. Non-rapid-eye-movement sleep (non-REM sleep or NREM sleep), rapid-eye-movement sleep (REM)
2. beta waves; high-frequency, low-amplitude activity; and sawtooth waves.
3. low, high
4. alpha waves (>50 percent)
5. rolling eye movements
6. high
7. light sleep stages, deep sleep or slow-wave
8. 75–80 percent
9. 3–8 percent, 40–45 percent, 15–20 percent
10. transitional
11. hypnic myoclonia
12. low-voltage, mixed-frequency activity, with alpha waves (8–12 Hz, <50 percent) and theta waves; beta waves (>13 Hz)
13. Vertex waves; rolling eye; decreased activity and muscle relaxation
14. light sleep stage
15. irregular, theta waves (4–7 Hz), sleep spindles, K complexes; Vertex waves
16. slow, absence of slow
17. low

18. decrease
19. 40 to 50 percent
20. 20 to 50 percent, high-amplitude (>75 μV), frequency (2 Hz or slower) delta waves
21. sleep spindles, K complexes
22. little or no eye movement, low
23. 50 percent, delta waves (amplitude >75 μV, and frequency 2 Hz or less)
24. no, little or no
25. 20 to 30
26. eyes open—wake state
27. low-voltage, mixed EEG activity; sawtooth waves; Alpha waves
28. REM
29. low electrical activity, paralysis
30. increases, decreases
31. increased, decreased
32. 25
33. 70 to 90, 5 to 30
34. restful; paradoxic sleep
35. dreams; vivid content, full color, sounds, implausible or bizarre settings, and a sense of paralysis

NORMAL SLEEP CYCLES

1. 10 to 30
2. sleep latency
3. 5, excessive
4. 30; lack of sleepiness, emotional stress, environmental disturbances, medication, illness, or pain
5. 1; 2, 3, and 4; 3 and 2; 2; REM; first sleep cycle
6. 2, sleep cycle
7. 90 to 110
8. longer
9. four and six
10. 30
11. 20 to 30
12. 5 to 30
13. increase, decreases
14. 1
15. stages 1, 2, and REM
16. REM
17. 20 to 40
18. awakenings
19. increase

FUNCTIONS OF SLEEP

1. restoration, energy conservation
2. restoration, recuperation
3. physical growth, healing; growth hormone

4. increased, proteins
5. attention span, learning and memory, emotional healing, and performance of basic social skills
6. homeotasis
7. 5 to 25 percent
8. declines

CIRCADIAN RHYTHMS

1. circadian rhythms
2. a. sleep–wake cycles
   b. changes in cortisol levels
   c. body temperature fluctuations
3. circadian synchronization
4. sleep debt

NORMAL SLEEP PATTERNS

1. few months
2. decrease
3. 16 to 17; seven
4. 3, 4
5. non-REM, REM
6. activity; twitching movements, gurgles, and coughing
7. 4
8. 14
9. 2, fifth
10. 8, 12
11. 8, 10
12. 6, 8
13. decrease, increases
14. 6
15. reduced or absent
16. longer

FACTORS AFFECTING SLEEP

1. a. age
   b. illness
   c. environment
   d. fatigue
   e. lifestyle
   f. emotional stress
   g. alcohol and stimulants

h. diet
i. smoking
j. motivation
k. medications

COMMON SLEEP DISORDERS

1. a. insomnia
   b. hypersomnia
   c. narcolepsy
   d. sleep apnea
   e. periodic limb movement disorder
   f. restless legs syndrome

NORMAL CARDIOPULMONARY PHYSIOLOGY DURING SLEEP

1. a. musculoskeletal system
   b. thermal regulation
   c. renal function
   d. genital function
   e. gastrointestinal function
   f. endocrine function
   g. cardiovascular function
   h. sleep-related arrhythmias
   i. cerebral blood flow
   j. respiratory physiology
2. paralyzed
3. obstructive sleep apnea
4. 1°C, 2°C
5. decreased, decreased
6. decreased
7. decreased, reduced
8. increases
9. decreased
10. sinusoidal
11. increased, decreased
12. heart rate, blood pressure, cardiac metabolism
13. heart rate and blood pressure, heart arrhythmias
14. decrease
15. increase
16. decreases
17. increases, decreases

CHAPTER EIGHTEEN

EXERCISE AND ITS EFFECTS ON THE CARDIOPULMONARY SYSTEM

EFFECTS OF EXERCISE

1. a. 20
   b. 3
   c. 6
   d. 25
   e. 20
   f. 20
2. 30, 60
3. 30, 50
4. 40
5. anaerobic threshold

VENTILATION

1. a. the cerebral cortex sending neural signals to the exercising muscles, which may also send collateral signals to the medulla oblongata to increase the rate and depth of breathing.
   b. proprioceptors in the moving muscles, tendons, and joints transmitting sensory signals via the spinal cord to the respiratory centers of the medulla.
   c. the increase in body temperature during exercise contributing to increased ventilation.
2. e
3. depth, rate
4. depth, frequency (rate)
5. f
6. a. an increase in alveolar ventilation, within seconds after the onset of exercise.
   b. a slow, gradual further increase in alveolar ventilation developing over approximately the first 3 minutes of exercise.
   c. alveolar ventilation stabilizes.
7. 50, 65
8. 250
9. 95
10. c

11. increased cardiac output
12. d

CIRCULATION

1. a. sympathetic discharge
   b. increase in cardiac output
   c. increase in arterial blood pressure
2. a. the heart is stimulated to increase its rate and strength of contraction
   b. the blood vessels of the peripheral vascular system constrict, except for the blood vessels of the working muscles, which dilate
3. an increased cardiac output
4. a. an increased stroke volume
   b. an increased heart rate
   c. a combination of both
5. vasodilation
6. Frank-Starling
7. 165
8. increases, decreases
9. a. the individual's physical condition
   b. the specific muscles that are working
   c. the distribution of blood flow
10. decreases
11. a. the sympathetic discharge
    b. the increased cardiac output
    c. the vasoconstriction of the blood vessels in the nonworking muscle areas
12. a. increases
    b. increases
    c. increases
    d. increases
13. local vasodilators

STROKE VOLUME VERSUS HEART RATE IN INCREASING CARDIAC OUTPUT

1. heart rate, increased stroke volume
2. 50
3. increased heart rate
4. 65

BODY TEMPERATURE/CUTANEOUS BLOOD FLOW RELATIONSHIP

1. profuse sweating, followed by no sweating; extreme weakness; muscle cramping; exhaustion; nausea; headache; dizziness; confusion; staggering gait; altered level of consciousness; unconsciousness; circulatory collapse
2. a. spraying cool water on the victim's body
   b. continually sponging the victim with cool water
   c. blowing air over the body with a strong fan
   d. a combination of all three

CARDIOPULMONARY REHABILITATION

1. a. the pretesting portion of the program
   b. patient and family education, group and individual counseling, and group discussion sessions
   c. follow-up care and long-term maintenance

CHAPTER NINETEEN

HIGH ALTITUDE AND ITS EFFECTS ON THE CARDIOPULMONARY SYSTEM

HIGH ALTITUDE

1. 18,000 to 19,000
2. increased alveolar ventilation
3. 6 weeks
4. c
5. c
6. 20 to 25 percent greater
7. a
8. increased
9. c
10. a

OTHER PHYSIOLOGIC CHANGES

1. a
2. headache, fatigue, dizziness, palpitation, nausea, loss of appetite, and insomnia.
3. second or third day after ascent.
4. vasoconstriction; increased
5. photophobia, ataxia, hallucinations, clouding of consciousness, coma, and possibly death.
6. fatigue, reduced exercise tolerance, headache, dizziness, somnolence, loss of mental acuity, marked polycythemia, and severe hypoxemia.

CHAPTER TWENTY

HIGH-PRESSURE ENVIRONMENTS AND THEIR EFFECTS ON THE CARDIOPULMONARY SYSTEM

DIVING

1. 1.0 atmosphere
2. a. 1.375 liters
   b. 3040 mm Hg (ref. Figure 20-1, pg. 554)
3. a. the diver's metabolic rate
   b. the diver's ability to store and transport O_2 and CO_2
4. 55
5. descends, ascends
6. hypoxia of ascent
7. a. bradycardia
   b. decreased cardiac output
   c. lactate accumulation in underperfused muscles
   d. peripheral vasoconstriction
8. a. joint pains (the bends)
   b. chest pain and coughing (the chokes)
   c. paresthesia and paralysis (spinal cord involvement)
   d. circulatory failure
   e. death (severe cases)

HYPERBARIC MEDICINE

1. (ref. Table 20-1, pg. 559)
2. a. increases the physically dissolved O_2 in the arterial blood
   b. increases the pressure gradient for driving oxygen into ischemic tissues
   c. reduces the half-life of carboxyhemoglobin (CO_{Hb})
3. 1 hour